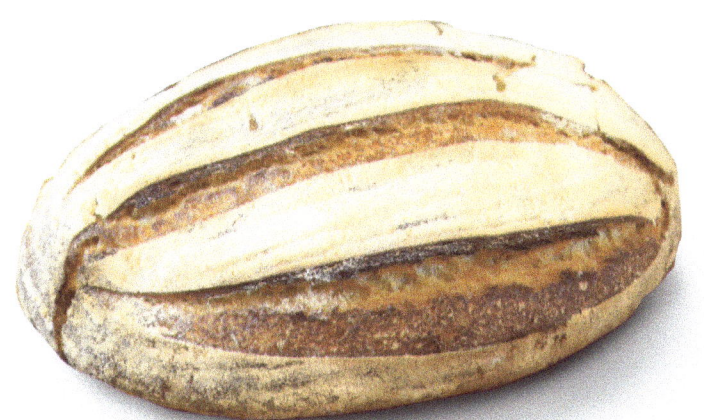

THE SOURDOUGH LOAF

By John Downes

Photography by Helen Carter

Additional photography / design by Mike Carroll

Published by Mike Carroll Media

9 Murtoa Rd, Eden Hills, South Australia, 5050

Copyright ©, Mike Carroll & John Downes, 2023

www.thesourdoughloaf.com

All rights reserved. No part of this publication may be reproduced, stored in a retrieval system or transmitted in any form or by any means, electronic, mechanical, photocopying, recording or otherwise, without the prior written permission of the copyright owner.

The moral rights of the author have been asserted.

ISBN: 978-0-6453496-0-3

Written by John Downes

Photography by Helen Carter & Mike Carroll

Design by Mike Carroll

Special thanks to Catherine Way

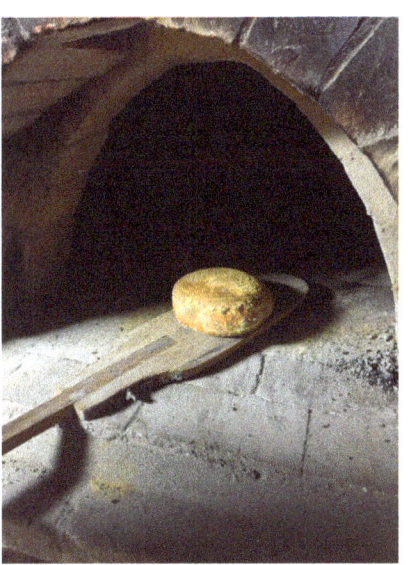

This book is dedicated to the memory of my son,
Sam Downes (Chimmers),

And to the late Lama Zopa Rinpoche.

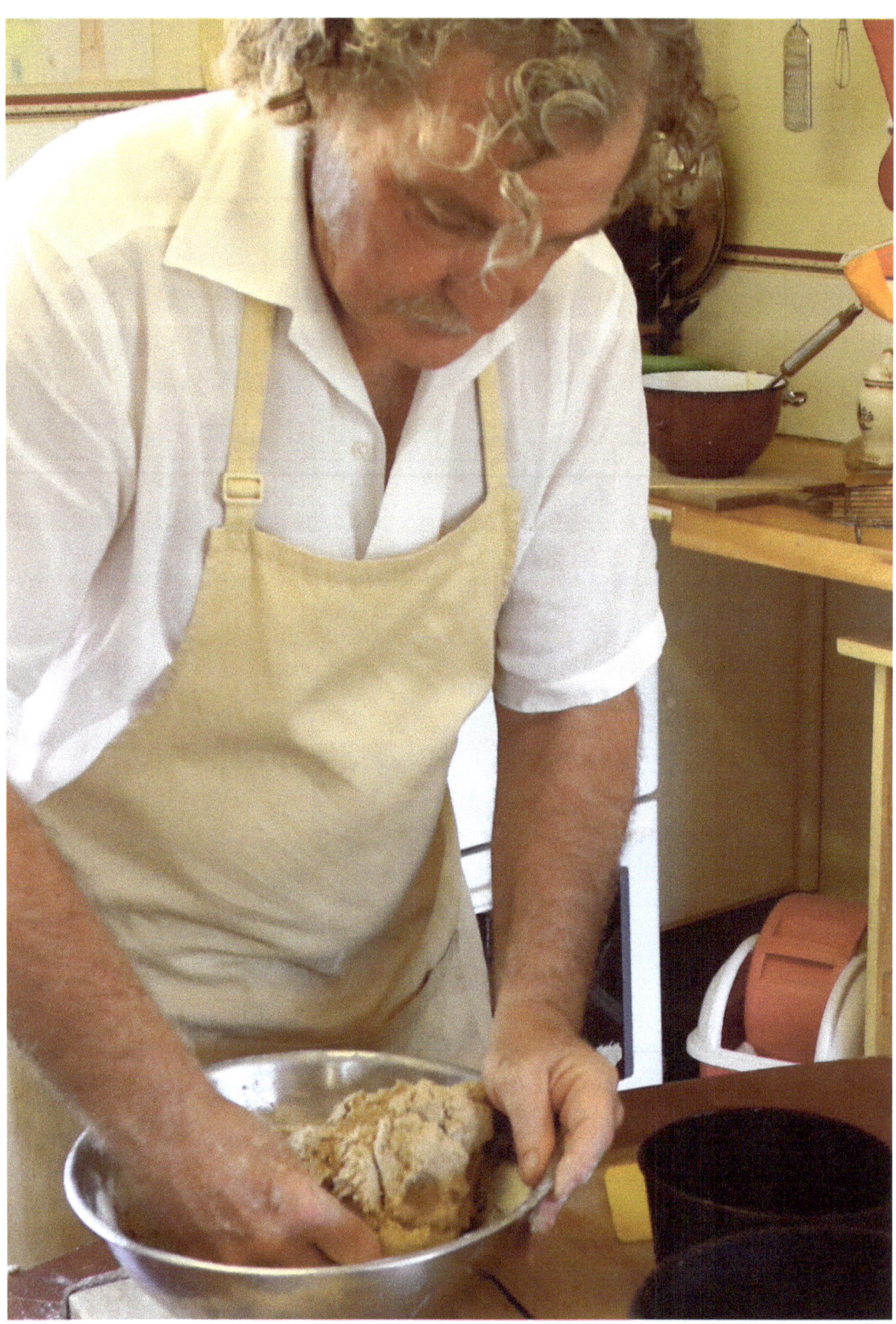

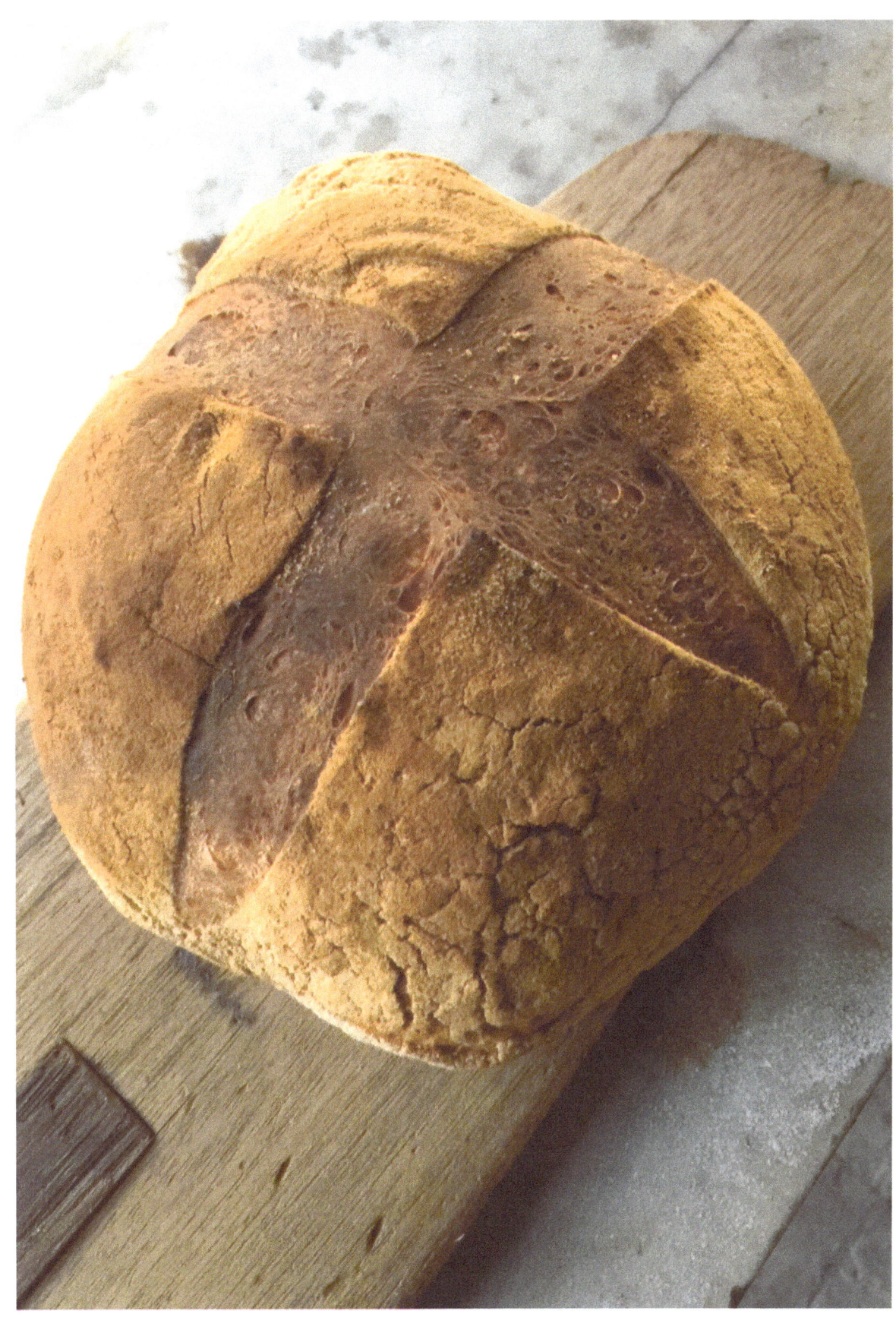

PREFACE.

Welcome. This is a conversational work for anybody interested in bread, food, cooking and their contexts, as well as a practical hands-on manual. The great English food author, Elizabeth David infected many of us with her background narrative, and certainly myself with her brilliant work "English bread and yeast cookery", and I scarcely laid it aside for over a year when it was first published. She gave license to "being there" in cooking - and to mildly rant. Much inspiration came from her book, which gave an order and confirmation to my experiences.

I started making bread in 1972, and subsequently stumbled upon the sourdough experience. Making the "Apple Cider Bread" (in recipe section) and later eating pretty damn sour "traditional" sourdough in San Francisco (Hy Lerner's wood-fired oven Flemish Desem bread in Boston, USA) was culinary Shaktipat - a spiritual awakening. The place of bread became clear; why bread is so often colloquially synonymous with virtually anything of value, notably money, but also in the tropes of Christianity and even the Sumerians. His bread was like a consecrated host, or Ayahuasca!

History and archaeology tell us the first farmers (not the band) ate "cereals and grains" - which makes little sense to a 'modern'. Porridge? Gruel? Really? Actually not: The Ancients made really good sourdough breads from their "cereals". There is an excellent National Geographic piece where Ed Wood recreates ancient Egyptian bread in an unearthed ancient Egyptian bakery, in the ancient Egyptian way. We didn't cover that at school or university, but without such visceral context it's all just academic.

On the every-day level, when made well, sourdough bread is just so good to eat - and eat with other simple foods. Dare I mention the ancient triad: bread, wine/beer/ale/cider and cheese? But also with last night's curry the next morning - I've seen many dinner parties taken over by a shimmering crusty sourdough seducing the diners with its charms and leaving the cheffy stuff paling.

Have the sourdough experience, be eaten alive.

-John Downes,
November 2021

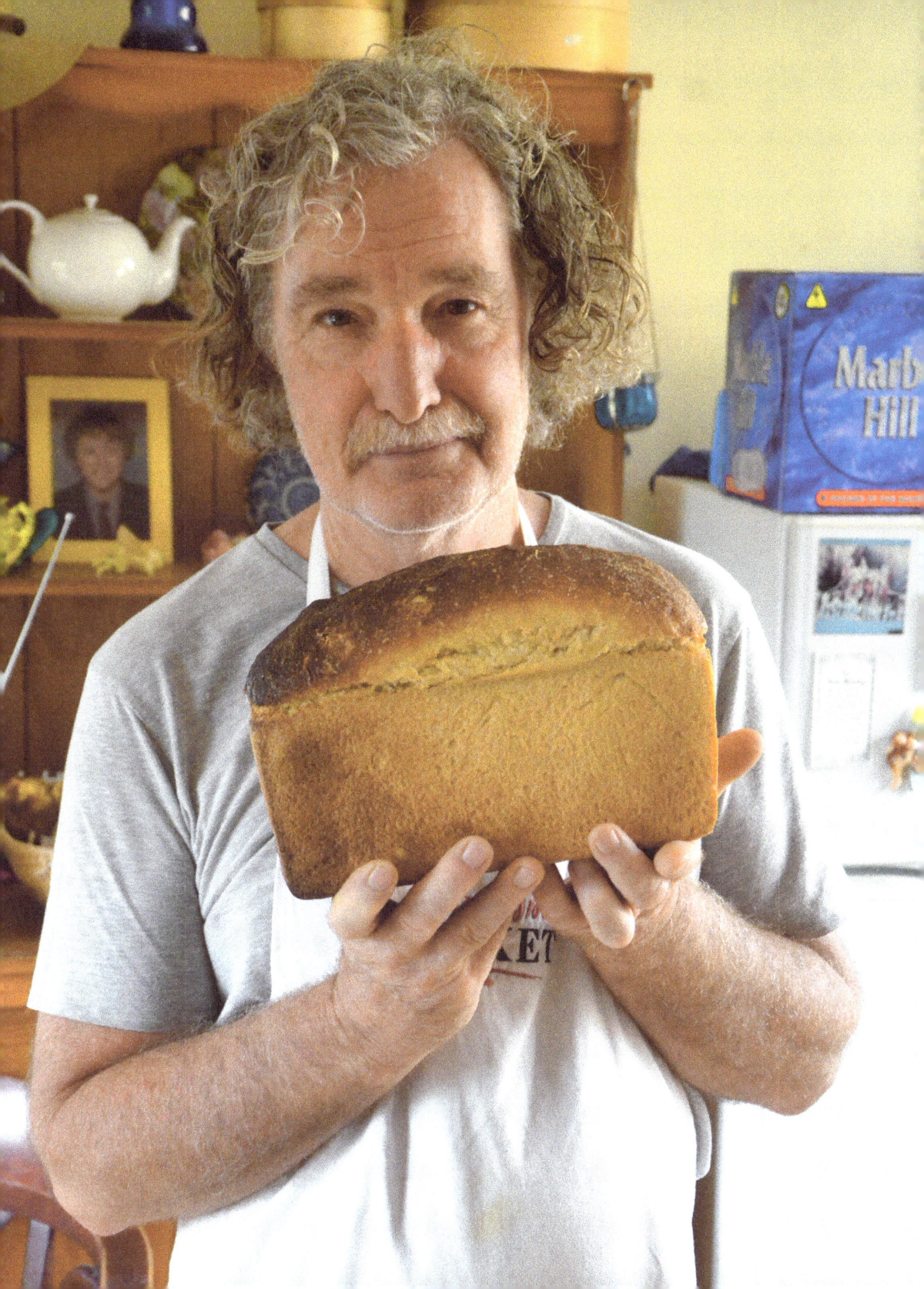

Table of Contents

Part 1.

Introduction	12
Why Bake Your Own?	17
Is Wheat Toxic?	21
Sourdough Fast Food	29
Ingredients	31
Stairway To Leaven	41
Dad's Wheat	51
Equipment For Baking.	57
The Oven	65
Techniques And The 4 Ts	69
Method For A Crusty Bread.	81
Method For A Tin Bread.	85

Part 2.

Crusty White Sourdough	91
Crusty Brown Bread	93
Boule	95
Panes Cum Toto	97
Crusty Chickpea Bread	101
Crusty Chestnut Bread	102
Great White	103
Corn Bread	105
Other "Corn" Breads	107
Pain De Campagne	109
Schwarzbrot	110
Crusty Spelt Bread	111
Emmer Bread	117
Emmer Flatbreads	119
Tropical Fruit Bread	120

Table of Contents Cont.

Barmbrack	121
Kuri Azuki Pan	125
Apple Cider Bread	127
Must Bread	131
Purple Wheat And Yellow Corn Bread	135
Rice Bread	137
Ginger Bread	139
Barm Bread	141
Bread Of The Rings	147
Barley And Oat Ring Breads	151
Wheat Ring Breads And Crumpets	152
Barley And Hazelnut Ring Bread	152
Finale Ring Bread	153
Buckwheat And Chestnut Ring Breads	154
Saffron Oatcakes	154
Muffyns	155
Socca: Chickpea Manna	159
Dhokla	162
Idli	163
Saffron Buns	167
Steam Buns	171
Steam Bread	171
Cacao Buns	173
Puri And Pufftaloons	175
Apple Sourdough	177
Brownies	178
Cheese And Onion Rolls	179
Crumble	181
Index	184

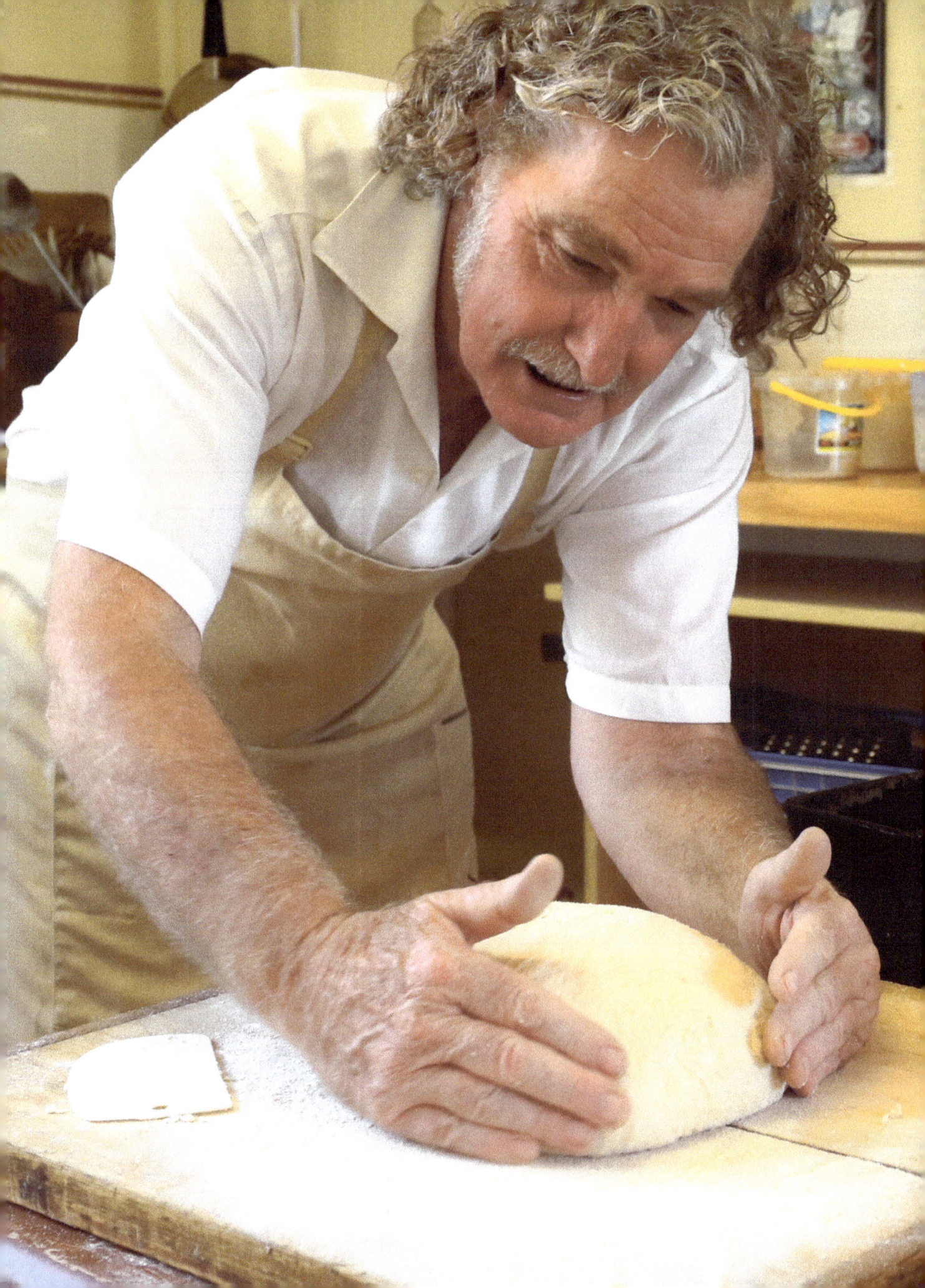

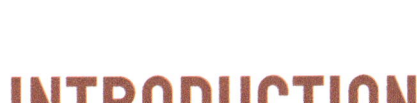

INTRODUCTION

Sourdough bread may seem novel, even hip, but in reality it is the way bread has been made forever, since the first mixture of flour and water. Sourdough bread has simply been lost in the mists of time as we romance the new, hygienically wrapped, soft white cuboid crumb, seemingly devised for space travel.

The idea that "bread" could be somehow central to so much seems ridiculous to 'moderns' thoroughly imprinted with an industrial archetype. Bread has changed so much that the collective racial memory of bread is virtually gone.

The present culinary zeitgeist is a curious mix of the future and the archaic, allowing sourdough bread to reveal itself again as the "bottom line" of food, the way to eat and digest the cereal grains we are urged to eat more of.

Sourdough bread actually is a force of nature, leavened or risen by natural or wild yeasts and benevolent bacteria. This symbiotic combination replaces the yeast generally used in bread making. These leavening agents are elemental in that they are components of the atmosphere as well as the grain itself.

It is easy to capture these elementals simply by leaving wholegrain flour and water as a batter, to ferment naturally without any human interference, apart from perhaps stirring, although even this is not necessary. Within days the batter is showing the classic signs of fermentation, bubbling and frothing with clear biological activity.

This active batter can then be mixed with more flour, water and salt (also an elemental), then allowed to continue to activate (rise) and finally be baked with fire (another elemental) to produce a very delicious well risen bread.

Such bread is clearly a gift of nature, is inherently "natural" and we are simply the conductors of this masterful synergy. Even more, we are a type of sourdough ourselves, as we are largely sustained from fermentation within our own personal biome.

Sourdough bread is both aesthetic and nutritional, a paradigm of culture. Made skilfully and if baked in a wood-fired oven, it is arguably the most difficult of the culinary skills, the most fundamental, and produces the most visceral associations from aroma to digestibility.

This bread is not yeast-free as often stated. It is simply free from the inbred and mono-cultured yeast which leavens most modern bread. The sourdough yeasts are a poly-culture, a multi-cultural society of different strains of yeast, while the bacteria are similarly complex and mostly from the lactobacillus tribe.

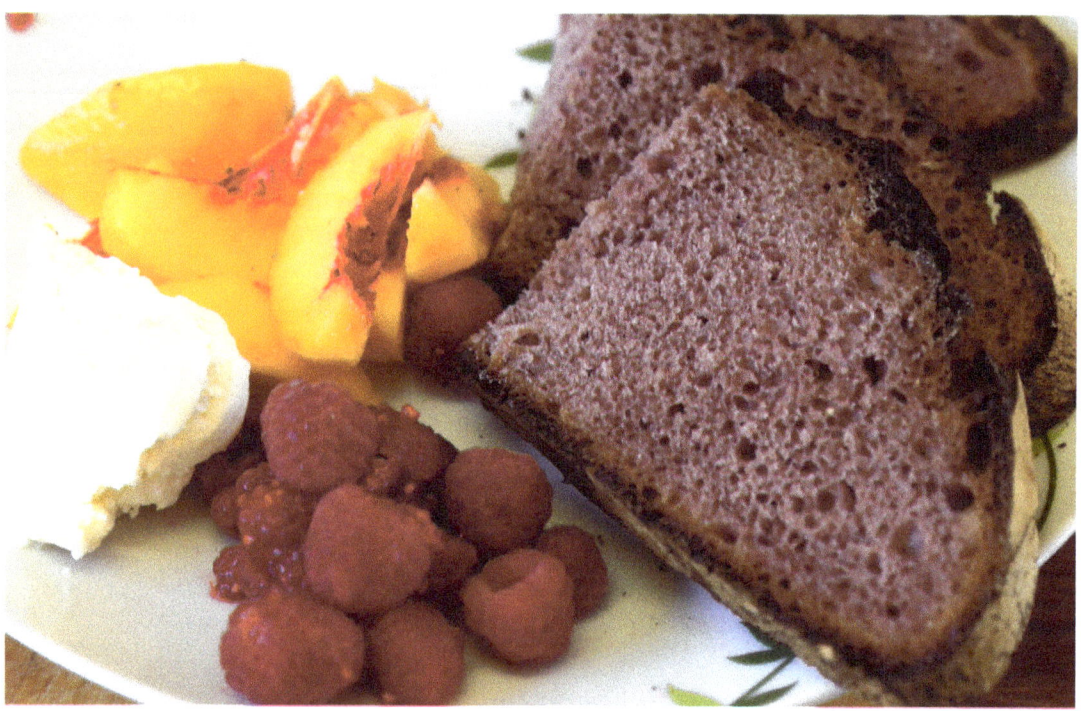

The cooperative action of these families of micro-organisms causes the rise or leavening of sourdough bread. They actually pre-digest the grain matrix rendering it highly digestible and the nutrients within the cereal bio-available, which means it eats well and is very nourishing.

New nutrients are also synthesised within the sourdough process, the bread being more nutritious than its original components. For example vitamin b12, necessary for life, has been found in my leavens in good quantity and this is unknown in regular bread.

Extra essential protein is also synthesised, which makes the protein component more balanced and significant as nutrition. Valuable minerals such as calcium and phosphorus, among others, are liberated from the complex structures which bind them within the cereal, also making the bread more nutritious than the grain from which it is made.

Organic acids and alcohol develop during the fermentation, considerably modifying the much maligned gluten proteins, rendering them more digestible. There is plenty of evidence that even coeliacs (those unable to digest the wheat protein gluten) can eat properly-made sourdough wheat bread, and that diabetics can benefit from it. As these both may arguably be conditions of "modernitis", the role of sourdough bread in modern life becomes more significant.

As a professional baker of sourdough bread for 45 years, I have noticed an almost viral phenomenon: the "magical" reversal of digestive complaints if proper sourdough replaces regular bread. It was almost like a zombie movie as folk stared longingly at my bread, enveloped by the heady aromas of the bakery only to tell me they could not eat bread for a variety of reasons. I always gave them a loaf to try, almost out of pity. Not one returned disappointed, rather being elated to eat bread again, with no symptoms, and delicious bread at that.

It is commonly thought that bread doesn't, even shouldn't, taste. Most peoples' experience is of factory bread is indeed that it does not taste, but nobody really knows, because such bread is usually simply swallowed. Chewing factory bread is actually a disaster as the wad so-formed is near impossible to swallow. It is raw gluten.

The texture of good sourdough bread is often called "dense", and compared to an airy supermarket loaf, this is accurate. The difference becomes apparent when one chews sourdough bread. In seconds, the seemingly dense crumb becomes creamy and smooth, as though the body accepts it and draws-in the nutrients. Moments later, the now creamy bite can be easily swallowed and again, the body seems to accept it with satisfaction.

Of course sourdough bread is "heavy" as by comparison, industrial bread is mostly air and water, yet this heaviness is merely a sign of good value, and it is light on the digestion.

Sourdough bread is surprising and complex in its flavour. "Sour" is in some ways an unfortunate label as the sour flavour is not widely appreciated and even suggests the unpleasant. The sour should be a lower profile of the flavour. Too much sour flavour in the bread is a fault, even though some do appreciate it. The sourness, acidity or "twang" (in old parlance) is from the bacterial component of the ferment becoming more dominant than the wild yeasts or the inherent flavour of the cereal.

The balance of flavours is the art of making and baking sourdough. The twang can also vary itself from the citrus-like mildness of more organic acids which form naturally in the ferment, to the vinegar-like (acetic) harshness of unskilled sourdough. No sourness at all is also from faulty technique and may betray an inauthentic sourdough, and there are plenty such imitations.

The flavour of wheat or grain should be dominant, liberated by the fermentation. This is gene-deep wheaten flavour, beyond "comfort", more "being". If the bread is crusty and burnished, as is desirable, the well-developed crust should infuse the inner grain flavours with wafts of roasted nuts, coffee, malt and cacao, depending on the skill of the baker, the grain itself, and the oven.

Few would deny that the redolence of a wood-fired sourdough loaf is incomparable, not simply smokey but fully enhanced by the elemental alchemy of the ferment, the fire and the heart. This is bread you can simply eat unadorned so good is the flavour, which also melds with and improves any topping.

It is surprising to moderns that sourdough bread was once common in Australia and England, the "Anglosphere", not simply in France, Europe and San Francisco. Many an "old-timer" has commented to me that "this is how bread used to taste", so recent is its fall from grace, almost hunted to extinction like so much wild-life.

Modern white factory bread is only 70 years old, yet has stamped generations with its imprint. Time is so fickle we now think of sourdough as "trendy", "new" or "fashionable", whereas in reality, these terms apply to white factory bread.

Bread, and here I mean sourdough in one form or another, was until recently the main food (staple) of most people. Other foods simply accompanied the bread. It had to be skilfully made, being the staple food, and was the preserve of trained artisans, members of the most important guild, or of the devoted family member. Today, the "other foods" dominate our meal with bread being relegated to sandwiches and the butt of jokes as "white tiles", "thongs", "white death" or even a signifier of cultural blandness, "white bread music", as well as the bane of the gluten intolerant, where once it was the centrepiece of religion, culture and economics.

One wonders if the apparent revival of sourdough bread as a major food is more than fashion, but an imperative, something elemental which has arisen from the depths of our humanity, reinforcing our human roots not as palaeolithic carnivores but in the fields of wild grain. Our anthropological niche is in reality, as the grass-seed eaters - "when a body meets a body, comin' thro' the rye".

Good bread is as worthy of restoration as the many other aspects of our past we are now learning to treasure.

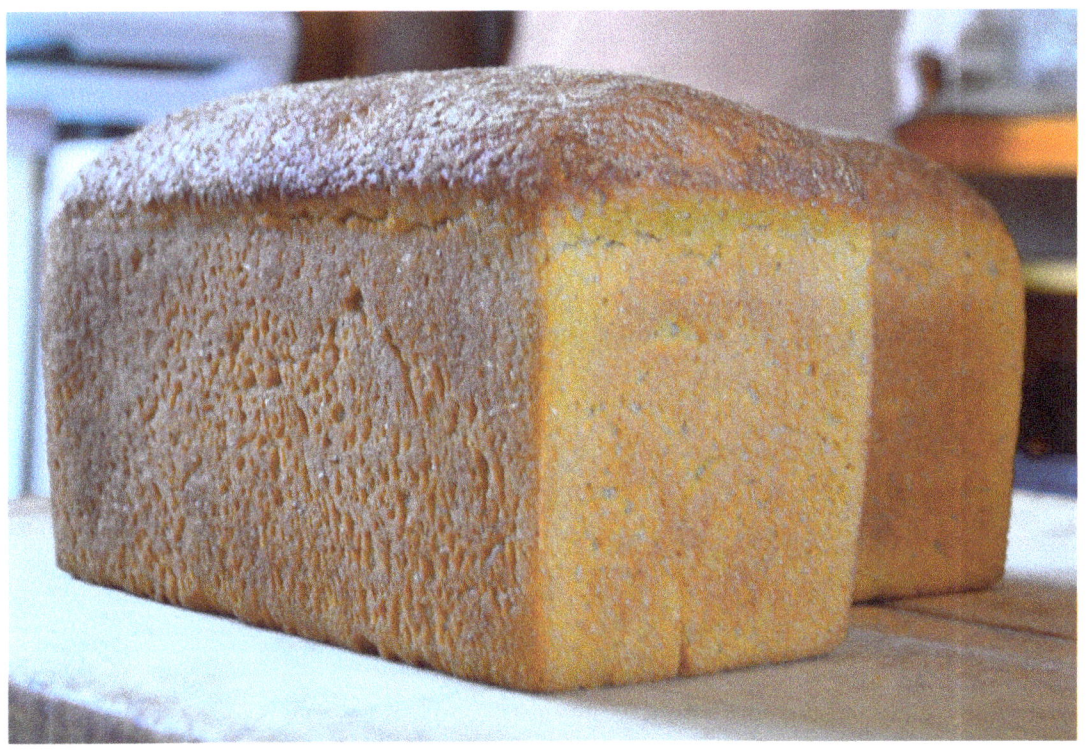

WHY BAKE YOUR OWN?

Choosing to bake your own bread is a powerful and empowering choice. It enables a degree of control over what you and yours eat, which is no small feat today. Apart from being a healthy choice it is also a gastronomic choice and these need not be separate.

Baking your own bread does not really consume much time, and can be an island in an ocean of emotion, apart from being a culinary triumph. More rewarding skilful and nourishing than making the "party food" we spend so much time creating and perhaps eating too much of.

Even though good sourdough bread is available in some areas, sourdough bread is not always what it seems. As there are no regulations governing the authenticity of sourdough, the makers/bakers are free to add whatever they like and often sourdough bread is simply yeast bread in the image of the real thing.

Hopefully you are lucky to have the real thing available. For those who don't have an authentic sourdough available, choosing to make your own is a rewarding choice.

Bread making/baking is often termed "therapeutic", an aspect much commented upon. Given the cultural/historical/gastronomic gravitas of sourdough as a food, making it creates a link, a portal to the time-honoured function which may well be a moderating factor on the "modernitis" which many feel. Even the rhythmic mixing or assembly of your bread kit may induce solace, as "culinary yoga", applied mindfulness.

This is different to regular bread making which utilises yeast. The sourdough journey is based on simpler, more elemental ingredients, one of which is time, the great moderator. Surrendering to the process which requires some of your precious time and attention can indeed be "therapeutic". At least you will have delicious bread, something tangible as a result of your efforts, which continues to feed-back as it is eaten, bestowing sunshine on your stomach.

Making sourdough bread is a method to approach well-being.

I once confided to a Tibetan Buddhist lama that I said mantras while I shaped hundreds of loaves of bread, which helped to maintain my focus, rather than being liturgical or an attempt at consecration. It is also in distinction to the violence with which dough is treated by some bakers. He burst out laughing thrilled at the idea of "blessed bread". This is certainly in keeping with a tradition with respect to bread, echoed in spirituality, which evokes wholeness. No matter if you do not share such convictions, the gastronomic quality of authentic sourdough bread is sufficient to command respect in its making, baking and eating.

Beyond bread baking being 'therapeutic" is the observation that hand-made bread, even commercially hand-made bread, involves a labyrinth-like ritual. Absently repetitive or mechanical, the bread is unsatisfactory, fails even. This aspect of ritual is paying attention to detail, being patient and present, a key to success in bread-making, revelatory even.

There is also a sense of satisfaction to be gained from sharing your bread, knowing that it bestows goodness to the young (especially hungry kids) and artistry to those aware. Such a sense of satisfaction can indeed be elusive and a treasure to find.

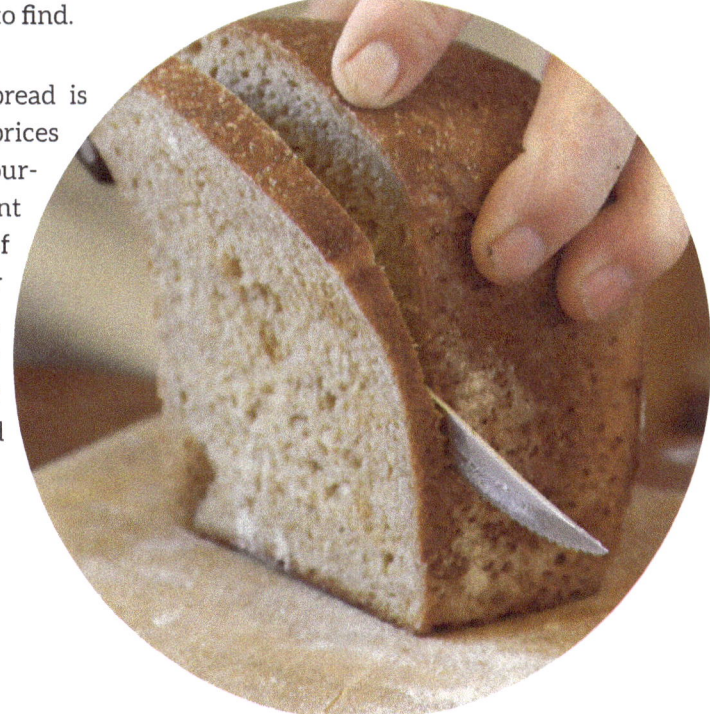

Making your own sourdough bread is also cost-effective as retail prices spiral. Apart from grinding-your-own, it is a worthwhile investment to purchase at least a 10kg bag of good flour from a miller or wholesaler as it will be fresher, retaining flavour. The good flour is then available to make other items, cakes pastries and savouries.

As nutrition "experts" flail around trying (unsuccessfully) to advise us about appropriate eating, the time-honoured tradition is to eat complex carbohydrates as the mainstay of your eating. As long as the "carbs" are from wholegrains, wholemeal, and your digestion works, nobody gets fat.

This is shown by the comparative health of those who eat this way, for example the "Mediterranean" diet, and the "Asian" diet. It is never mentioned that the basis of the Mediterranean diet is bread, usually sourdough but at least fermented to some extent, even with yeast. It is not olive oil, which is merely a condiment. Have you noticed there are (were) very few fat people in Asia, yet rice, even white is the staple food? Complex "carbs" do not make one fat.

The only people with major pathologies from diet are in the "west". It is called the "Western Pattern Diet", WPD, and it's in a store near you.

Eating sourdough bread is the culinary answer to the exhortations to eat "whole-grains". Most people have no idea what "wholegrains" are and how to eat them, and "cereal" has come to mean a crispy sugary thing for breakfast, an Orwellian linguistic victory for Big Food.

The "carbs" have to come from a correct source and sourdough bread is ideal. All unfermented regular bread, even the "healthy" ones, are a part of WPD. Those "multi-grain" loaves are dyed-pretty factory bread with dried grains added, which pass unchanged through the digestive tract and are merely eliminated.

Sourdough bread is the basis of a tried and true tradition, no need for a "study" on this, it has already been done.

Make and eat the life-giving bread.

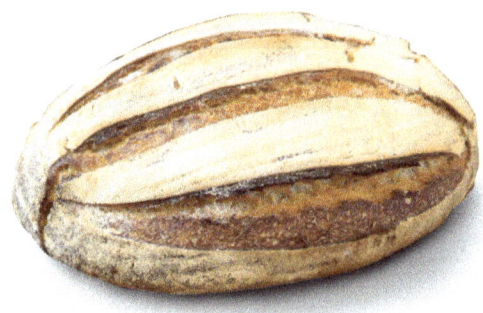

The Sourdough Loaf

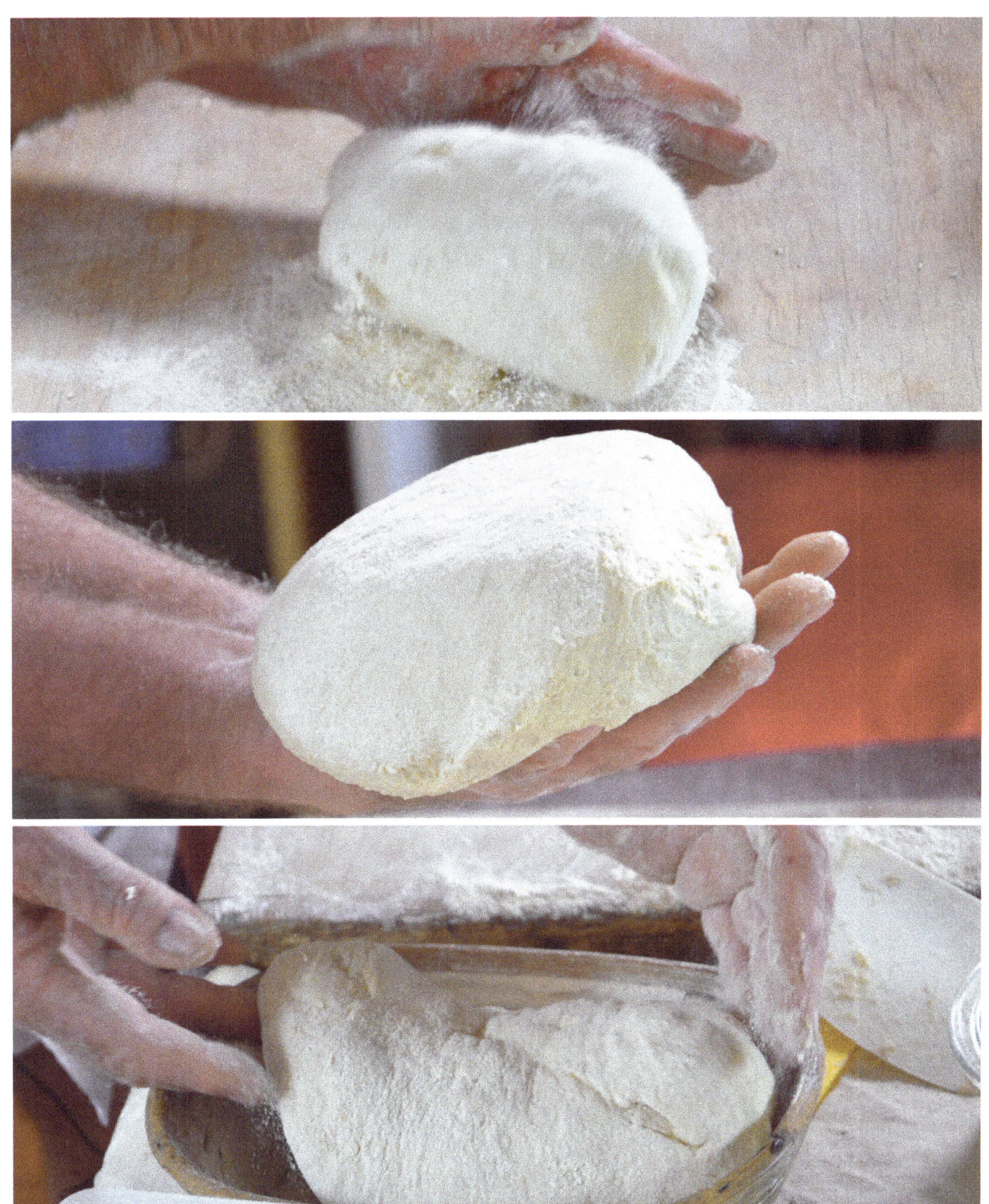

The Sourdough Loaf

IS WHEAT TOXIC?
(THE FLOUR SCENE FROM "PSYCHO")

Given the hype and rhetoric it would seem our spinning blue ball is experiencing a bout of the wheat blues. Gluten is the major protein in wheat, and apparently a growing number are "allergic " or reactive to a fraction of the gluten protein, its evil twin, gliadin.

Others seem to have a sensitivity to wheat itself. Gluten-free products are everywhere as are gluten-free options in eateries.

Many report feeling better since eliminating wheat, gluten, from their eating. Others are saying, "how can it be?", we have been eating wheat forever. The grumpy responses from the gluten cynics are entertaining. Even psychologists are onboard, quoting "confirmation bias". The latest is that it is "caused by a virus", and how many times have we heard that to explain almost any malady today?

We can be deeply grumpy about food.

Gluten intolerance.

Unfortunately for the "gluten-doubters" it seems that approximately one third of "Indo-Europeans", excluding east Asians and sub-saharan Africans, have the required genetic haplotype which pre-disposes us to a reaction to wheat gluten/gliadin. The highest frequency is in Europeans. This would appear to roughly correlate with those in society who are going gluten free. So be kind!

Clinical immune-reaction to gluten/gliadin is called coeliac disease and affects about 3-6 % of the population of western Europe and the USA as well as the "Anglosphere". It also affects the major wheat-eating nations from north Africa to India.

There are a few forms of wheat and gluten/gliadin intolerance and or allergy, and it is thought that some form of reaction to wheat and or fractions of it is more widespread than previously thought. The true prevalence may be higher than that estimated clinically, as screening studies using antibody testing have suggested there is a significant frequency of asymptomatic (silent) coeliac disease in the general population" according to gastroenterologist researchers in Sydney*.

There are varied symptoms of these wheat reactions, but the "common underlying immune pathogenesis is increased intestinal permeability*", but other researchers claim coeliac and others reactions to wheat have a "tremendously varied clinical presentation*"…very unhappy tummy, and all that leads from it, including neurological symptoms.

Clinically it is coeliac disease, but practically it is a reaction brought on by industrial white bread. This is where the massive doses of gluten started being eaten. There is no coeliac disease without gluten.

Bread for Coeliacs.

Trials in Italy have shown that fully-fermented sourdough can be eaten by coeliacs, and this is my experience as well. Unfortunately, there are very few fully fermented sourdoughs available commercially, and some bakeries and millers add still more gluten to flour, even to organic flour and to bread. Adding ascorbic acid as a dough "improver", as many do, actually preserves the gluten as well, preventing the sourdough (proteolytic or protein-cracking) enzymes from doing their important de-tox work.

In 40 years of baking genuine fully-fermented sourdough bread, eaten by many clinical coeliacs, with no adverse reaction whatever, and by others with NCGS (non-coeliac gluten sensitivity) also with no reactions, there is simply joy at being able to eat bread again.

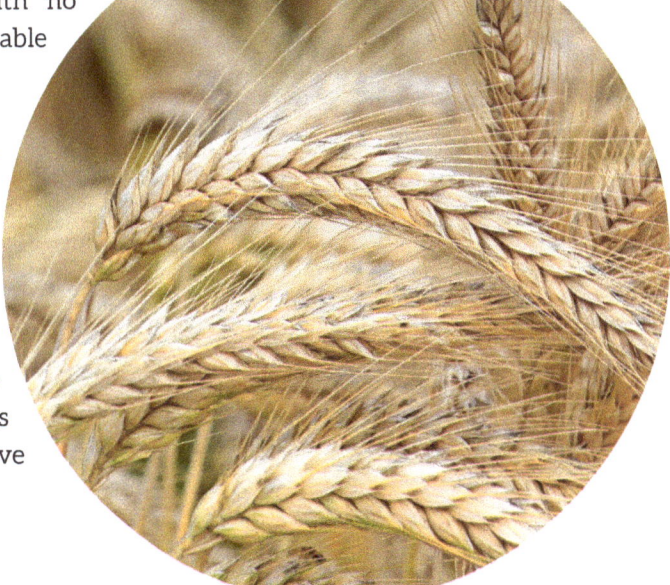

Most dried grains, and legumes especially, have a degree of "toxicity", as do potatoes. Legumes usually contain a trypsin (digestive enzyme) inhibitor which interferes with digestion, or some such bio-weaponary, to deter predators. Mice die if they eat dried legumes such as lentils because of these anti-nutritive inhibitors.

Corn, (maize) beloved of the "corn people" the native Americans, and now contemporary Americans, also contains a vitamin B inhibitor which is effectively toxic. This causes pellagra, inability to absorb B vitamins which devastated the American south and southern Europe until it was realised that the Indigenous American people always soaked the corn in wood ash/ lye water to remove this inhibitor. This is called "nixtimal-ising" an ancient code.

Soya beans must be well-soaked and cooked, sprouted or fermented to remove their "toxic" inhibitor, yet they are the "meat of the fields" for billions.

Potatoes if green, will not ripen, as I have heard, but should be shunned as this is a concentration of the poisonous alkaloid solanine. One writer commented that we each eat enough solanine in one year, which if given in a single dose, would kill a horse.

The gluten protein in wheat , or its gliadin fractions can be viewed the same way. The traditional method to render it harmless is to ferment it, as in sourdough bread.

Chorleywood "Wonder Bread".

When bread started being made commercially with yeast, which was approximately the 1880s, fermentation of bread was greatly reduced, and by the 1950s, eliminated altogether in the Chorleywood one hour wonder bread process, which is the factory bread most people eat today.

Notably the Chorleywood process employs a lot of added raw gluten as superstructure to maintain its high-rise.

The raw gluten is washed out of wheat flour. It is then dried and can be added as a powder or flour. The great boon for those seeking to monetise bread was that gluten absorbs double its weight in water, and because of its character as a polymer, when whipped at high speed with water, produces chains or long rope-like structures which are very tough.

This is similar to the tempering of metal to make high quality steel for a sword. The metal is beaten and folded and beaten and folded continually until it acquires a whole new, hard but flexible, stronger characteristic.

Consequently less flour and more water could be added, water being cheap, as is raw gluten. Using chemical bread "improvers" like ascorbic acid, makes the gluten tougher still, and resistant even to fermentation. Elizabeth David in "English bread and yeast cookery" called it "solidified water".

A recipe for disaster, this heavily developed gluten is not readily digestible, and is seemingly designed to resist breakdown through digestion. Machines replaced hands and chemists replaced bakers.

The next step in the disastrous industrialisation of bread, was to preserve the gluten from fermentation even more, by using highly selected and modified yeasts which like to feed on the added refined sugar, reproduce rapidly, produce very little acid to breakdown the gluten, and make a lot of gas to be trapped in the super-tough gluten balloons, the airbags which we know as the texture of bread.

We started eating quite a lot of raw gluten, a first in the history of wheat and food, and this helps to explain why so many seem to react to bread in particular.

At least the brown and wholemeal flours eaten in the pre-refining past reduced the percentage of gluten in flour, but refining it to whiteness actually increased the amount of gluten as a percentage. White flour wasn't available at all until the 1860s unless one was a potentate of some variety and had their flour sifted through silk.

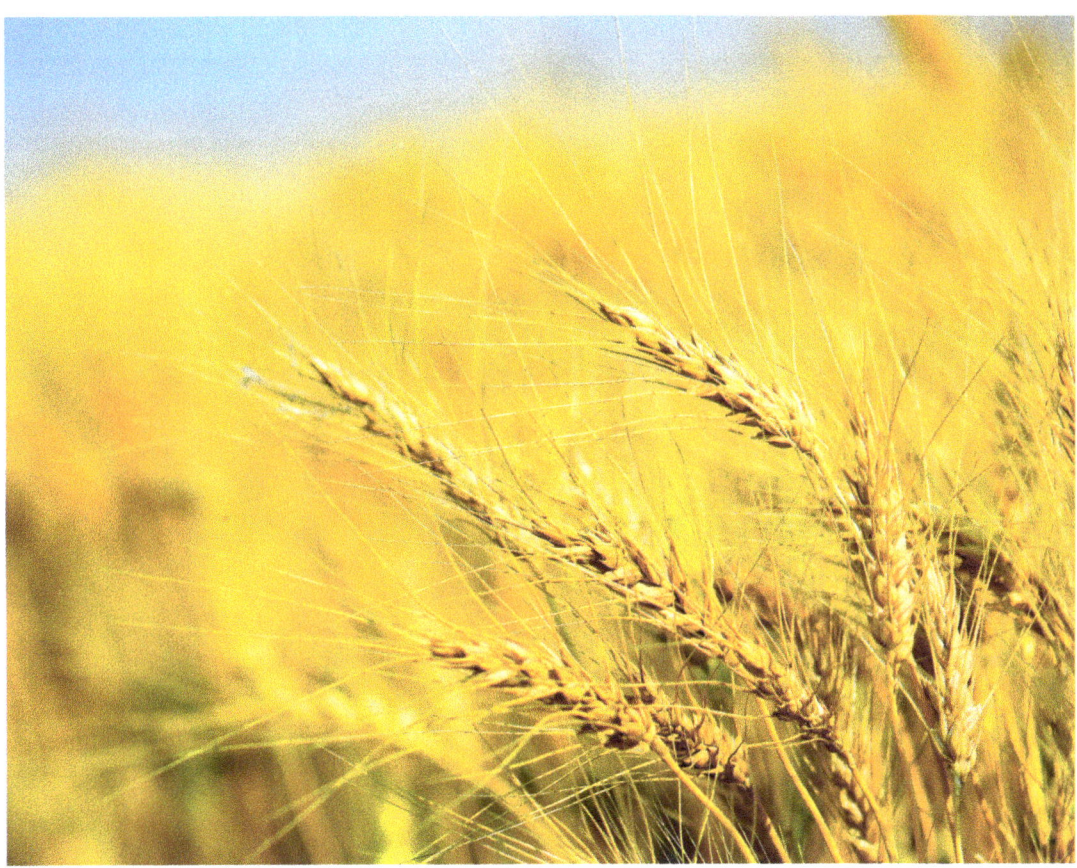

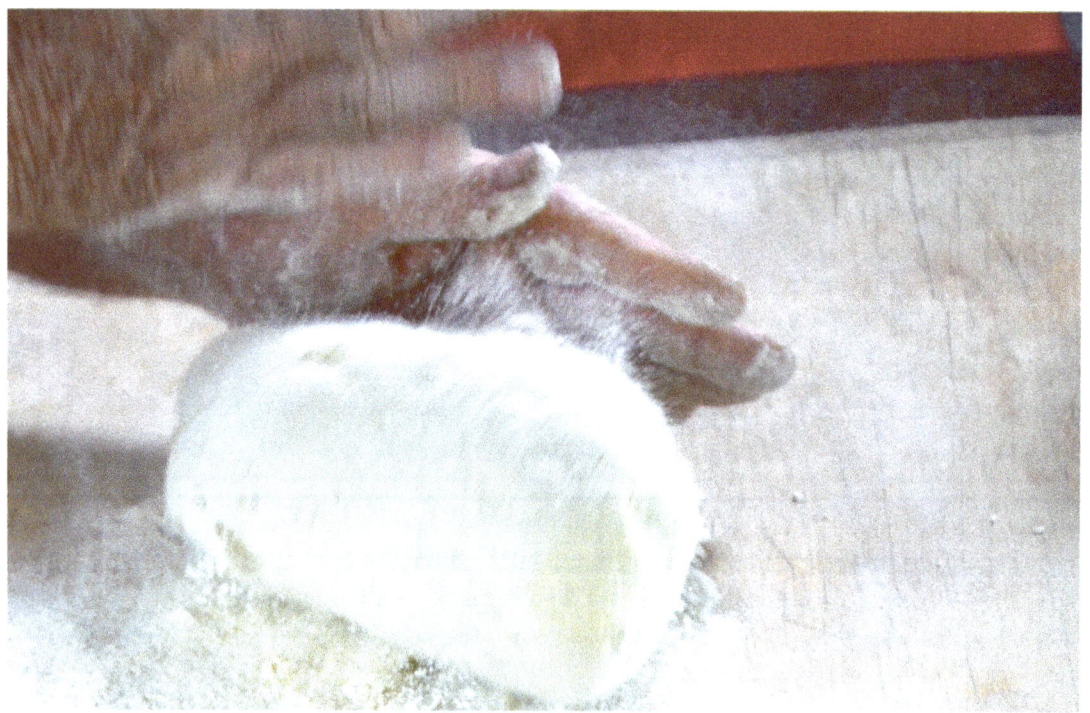

Wheat gluten is not soluble in water at all, but is soluble in acids and alcohol, which is largely why people have trouble digesting it. The sourdough process through its myriad bacteria produces organic acids and alcohol, both capable of breaking down gluten.

Given a historical perspective it is not surprising that 'moderns' exhibit various reactions to wheat. Add-in the well-known depletion of bowel flora from the WPD (Western pattern diet), antibiotic abuse and low stomach acid (a-chlorhydria), both symptoms of the WPD, and the demise of acidic and alcoholic condiments which break-down gluten, then couple that with the industrial doses of raw gluten we have suddenly been subject to, and an intolerance to wheat is actually to be expected. It's almost a dietetic trial, played out epigenetically, as coeliacs can pass on this acquired condition to 1/3 of their offspring.

The coeliac's solution? Best make your own sourdough bread, unless blessed with a baker who cares and knows - and they do exist.

We've *always* eaten wheat.

It is also not accurate to claim that 'we have eaten wheat forever so how could this be? Wheat was of course eaten in central and western Asia where it grew wild, but in temperate areas wheat was only eaten by those who could afford it.

Wheat was the preserve of the wealthy. In the UK for example, the English nobility ate "manchet", made from sifted wheat flour and risen with barm yeast. This was entirely different to the traditional yeoman's loaf, the English pain de campagne, which was a sourdough made with a minimum of wheat and depending on the season, mixed with rye, barley, buckwheat, oats, legumes, chestnuts, hazelnuts, acorns, or even dock seeds. The term "bread" has a very wide sweep.

In Ayurvedic medicine, the traditional medicine of India and central Asia, wheat is regarded as potentially toxic to a certain body-type, the "kapha" type. Interestingly, in line with now-revealed genetic markers, approximately one-third of the population are predominantly "kapha" types. Known to put on weight easily, in Ayurvedic dietetics they have traditionally been advised to avoid or minimise wheat. This shows the "modern" problem was historically well known, and indicates its potentiality, demonstrating that we dismiss traditional proto-scientific knowledge of food and dietetics to our peril.

Apart from the gluten added to bread and other foods, wheat gluten has changed considerably in the past 150 years. New wheat strains began to appear in the late 1800s largely from Canada where a chance planting of a few seeds of Ukrainian hard wheat produced dramatic results.

These Canadian hard wheats caused a sensation in the UK in the late 1800s where it was noted that the same weight of flour as normally used, required more water than "home" wheat, but resulted in an extra loaf than was usual from the mix! These hard wheat flours were much in demand and allowed the development of the "French" bread (actually Viennese) now widely made and praised.

The wheat breeders went to work and slowly developed harder wheats. The famous "red fife" wheat from Canada was a progenitor of many new strains. What the plant breeders did in their search for stronger wheat, was to increase the gliadin fraction in wheat, seemingly toughening-up the gluten, thus increasing the allergenic part of the gluten molecule.

The ancient wheat Emmer has in fact more protein than modern wheat, but modern wheat has an exaggerated "glia-alpha 9 sequence", according to some, making it far more allergenic. Emmer has very little gluten, let alone gliadin. The proteins in heirloom wheat, apart from being in greater quantity than modern wheat, were the water soluble proteins, easy to digest, and many of these were bred-out in favour of the gluten protein.

Recently, genetic material from dwarf wheat was introduced widely, and modern industrial wheat is merely knee-high to suit mechanical harvesting. It was not uncommon for heirloom wheat to be human-height and even taller. This again has changed the character of wheat in the genetic-shuffle, and codes for flavour and "bloom" appear to be lost. The plant breeders also bred the flavour out of wheat, as heirloom strains are quite dramatically full-flavoured compared to the "cardboardy" hard wheat now favoured, and often produced a more colourful crust "bloom" - once much sought after.

Much of this is contentious, as others argue that wheat germ agglutinin, a different fraction of wheat, is also allergenic, or that the glyphosate now routinely sprayed on harvested wheat grains to "condition" them causes intestinal irritation mimicking coeliac symptoms.

What seems observable to me as a baker of 40 years, talking to many customers, usually about their "wheat problem", is that nobody has a digestive issue with properly fermented sourdough bread. The fermentation creates a highly nutritious and well-accepted food.

Some bakers and "breadsmiths" know only too well that the old wheats like spelt or khorassan or heirlooms are much more difficult to bake with as the fermentation times are very critical. Modern wheat allows the baker to walk away and have a cuppa, but the heirloom wheat demands full attention as it is observably much less "strong". The new wheat clearly contains a lot more gluten, and more robust gluten at that.

It is worth using "soft" and cake-wheat flour, or spelt, khorassan or emmer wheat, and make fully-fermented traditional flatbreads, and only wholemeal, if to you, wheat seems hard to digest. By chewing well, using traditional acidic or alcoholic condiments, drinking good wine or cider or ale when the meal includes wheat or bread, wheat may become more tolerable for those in need. The "bread and wine" culinary/religious meme is well attested.

If you really don't want to eat wheat, use the recipes for Soca (chickpea flatbreads) to make delicious sourdough or explore the tasty rice bread recipe.

*A major source : Current Therapeutics, June 1998..."Coeliac Disease" by Selby and Faulkner Hogg.

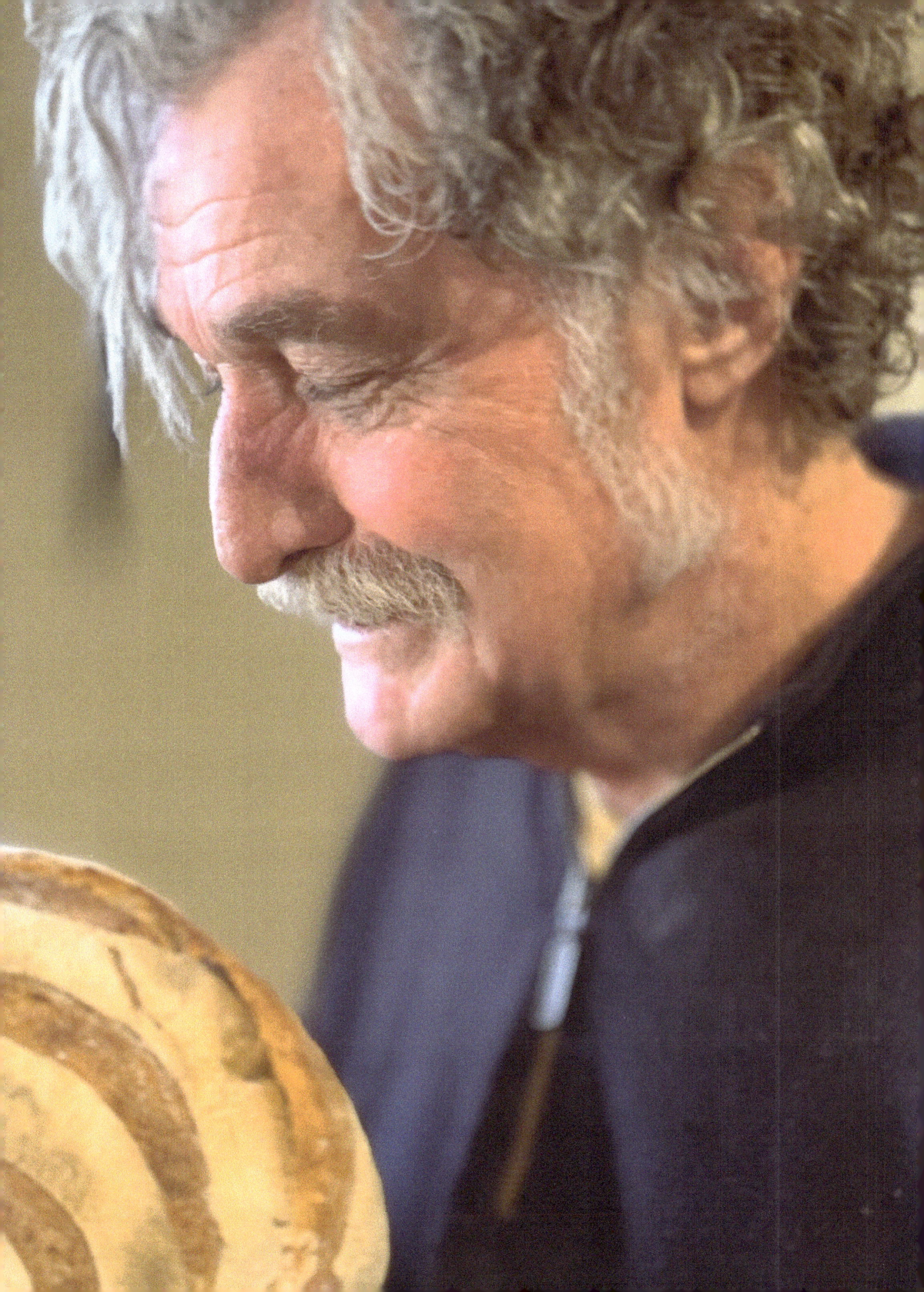

SOURDOUGH FAST FOOD

Buried within the fast food world is the original fast food, but now made in factories, packed with preservatives and clever (dishonest) techniques and labelling. The white cuboid crumb, largely devoid of nutrients, except for those added back in to replace the ones refined out, is there, always there - but not as popular as it once was.

Until the current "real" bread revival, bread consumption had declined dramatically, even when we were given what the industry claimed we wanted (it was wheat "they" wanted) — the *Chorleywood process* bread which was pure in colour (white), soft as cake, tasteless, and required no chewing. It sounds like water really, which it largely is, except it is not odourless, it has the mysterious aroma of factory bread, which is not the aroma of grain, nor is it the actual aroma of bread.

Walking down that bread aisle in a supermarket, I struggled to establish an analog aroma. Although it made me nauseous trying to plumb the mysterious aroma of factory bread, I gave up because it is a chemical smell and has no analog in the natural world, although it is strangely close to the smell of wet old hessian bags.

When the first wave of post WW2 immigrants came to Australia when I was a lad, it astonished me that some of my European school friends would eat a piece of bread unadorned with the camouflage we used. As commented upon elsewhere, white factory bread cannot be chewed and cannot (is never) eaten without some, any, topping. But the bread they were eating was not white factory bread, it was different. My mother called it "continental bread", which considering we lived in Australia was incomprehensible to me. But we both had our fast food.

This dovetailed nicely with my innocent disbelief at the "last supper", with Christ breaking bread and it being shared - without butter, vegemite, jam or marmite. Impossible!

Bread has always been "fast", and once made is an easily accessed instant food of great convenience, requiring no further fuss or cooking and was inherently nutritious.

This is where we enter the world of simulacra, because "fast" it still is, but no longer digestible and not really nutritious as the grain is now stripped of its goodness and is moulded into a whiter than white image of food, a mere statue of the deity, to presage today's culinary dissonance; our simultaneous obesity and starvation.

Making sourdough bread, stocking your larder or freezing it, returns a hard-won convenience complete with its gastronomic and nutritional origins. Any sandwich whether open or closed becomes food again with sourdough bread. The flavour of the bread melds with and accentuates any filling or topping.

Ordinary toast becomes a worthy meal especially when we open up to traditional specialities such as bruschetta (Italian toast). We now have a canvas on which to compose modern portraits of global fusion and harmony, never before enjoyed and only genuine sourdough has the texture required to make a real bruschetta. In the garlic version, the raw garlic is rubbed into the freshly toasted bread, which is often less than ideal on regular bread, whereas the texture of sourdough rasps and holds a good quantity of garlic which is essential for the success of this dish.

Sourdough toast, rubbed with garlic, spread with good butter or olive oil topped with avocado, and or sweet heritage tomatoes, or any or all of, roasted pumpkin, olives, eggs, cheese, meats, or smashed peas, all invite culinary fusion and combinations of flavour to rival "picture on plates" - and it happens in minutes. How fast can food be? And with this wholesome bread, more immediate than waiting for (gastronomic) Godot.

Hunger is assuaged in seconds with good bread, and with satisfaction. Sourdough bread is the original fast food of which one does not tire and which is actually "food" rather than being "food-like", "the marrow of humanity" and a cornerstone of good, and even *fast* eating.

INGREDIENTS
The flowers of flour.

There are only three ingredients necessary to make genuine sourdough bread: flour, water and salt. This is alchemy between three elemental ingredients. The final element is the fire which bakes the bread.

Using the best possible ingredients stands to reason. Sourdough bread is a fundamental food which needs to be good to support health and well-being as well as its gastronomic quality and context. The best ingredients have premium flavour and potentially give the best results.

Flour is clearly the most important ingredient. Flour from wheat varies considerably and this variation can cause the most difficulty for any baker. Some will not have easy access to the most suitable flour for bread making, although now it can be ordered online. It is worth the effort to procure good flour, however you do it.

Types of Wheat.

There are basically two types of wheat, the harder (stronger) and the softer (weaker), although modern breeding and loss of heritage strains has muddied the waters somewhat.

Strong or hard wheat means strong flour which has the highest gluten content or muscle, and such flour will give the most stable dough and the highest, biggest rise. Strong flour doesn't have the best flavour, however, and the ideal flour is of medium strength, as in the classical heritage wheats.

Soft and hard flour have a very different feel. Good cake makers always sift their flour. They have to. Cake flour is soft and forms clumps easily. It feels talc-like.

Hard wheat bread flour is more gritty, sandy and is less easy to clump.

Soft wheat flour is almost always paler and whiter, as are its seeds, plump and yellow.

Hard wheat tends to be darker, glassy or flinty. There are variations however.

Soft wheat tends to have more essential wheaten flavour, biscuity even, the dominant flavour of authentic scones.

Blending a little soft flour with hard flour considerably improves bread flavour.

Soft wheat has a much lower gluten content and is used commercially for biscuits cakes and pastry. In skilful hands, soft wheat does make very flavoursome bread. A flour "rep" - a representative from a major flour company - reacted with animated horror when he discovered I was using their soft, cake flour for crusty breads. There was no margin for error, but the flour was so well-flavoured that it gave the best crust. Of course the bread wasn't an architectural wonder, but it had melt-in-the-mouth flavour.

Most people will simply shop for "flour" and fortunately some producers label their flour as suitable for bread-making or as "cake" flour. Modern, strong bread flour will give the best architecture/structure, nice sized loaves and potentially a fashionable lacy/holey, "alveolated" structure.

This sort of high-rise structure is a modern phenomena, a trend, but not necessarily the "best" bread. We are now imprinted with this sort of bread architecture from fashionable loaves, and the high-rise from factory bread. These well-built loaves are often made from patent flours containing added gluten which is difficult to digest or from inordinately strong flour.

Wheat Flours.

Flour varies around the globe and will absorb more or less water than stated in the recipes. For example Canadian hard wheat flour may require quite a bit more water than soft English flour, and this less than medium-strength Australian flour. When I first worked in the UK I looked on in dismay as one of my prize recipes turned to near soup because the flour was so much softer having a higher moisture content than flour I had used in Australia. It simply did not absorb as much water.

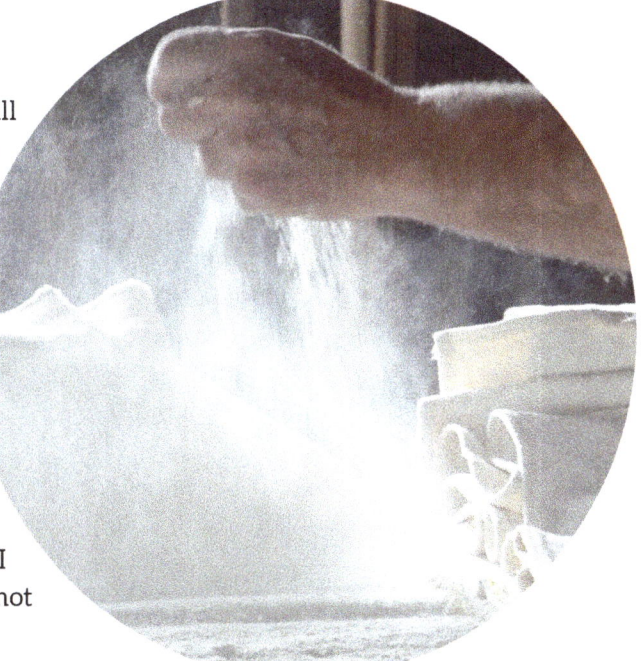

The Sourdough Loaf

It seems simplistic, but If the dough is too dry/hard/stiff/unyielding, add more water. If the dough is too soft/wet, add more flour.

It is the "feel" we have to learn and no recipe for sourdough bread can be exact, which makes genuine sourdough bread less mechanical and more informing and encouraging of our senses and skills. It also provides variation as your loaves will be different, all of our loaves will be different, whereas the common choice is for tired uniformity. It is also a taste of history as once we had bakers who made characteristic loaves, not the same as their rivals, and bread varied a lot.

If you cannot access ideal bread flour, consider making flat or flatter breads or bread of the rings (see recipes section). In some ways, flatbreads are the best choice for many. Flat breads are crusty yet with a pleasing soft interior texture and are a lot less fuss with a great margin of error. They are also the most historic/archaic and were originally baked "in the ashes".

Ideally, flour needs to be stone-ground from organic or biodynamic wheat. Other types of milling such as metal-burr mills are also superior, as the whole of the grain is crushed, dispersing inherent factors.

The practice of biodynamics, while arcane, even weird to some, nourishes the soil, is responsible, sustainable, and does make sense. The proof is that biodynamic flours are the most bio-active, producing the best leavens and the most flavoursome colourful breads, not to mention higher nutritional value, as biodynamic and organic wheat have extensive root structures which glean more nutrients from the enhanced soil. Conventional flour will work well, no doubt, but if you seek quality, source biodynamic or organic flour.

Most biodynamic and often organic flour, is stoneground. I have experimented for many years and have no doubt that stoneground flour is superior, also verified by analysis which shows that the valuable wheat germ oils and bran flavours infuse the whole flour during the slow grinding process. Clearly, this enhances the flavour and also the "bloom" or colour and aesthetic appeal of the bread.

Regular white flour (unbleached) is roller-milled, which means the wheat is ripped apart by steel teeth, and then finely sieved producing the white flour so craved yet perhaps so craven. It is no secret that this type of flour is at the root of dietary dysfunction. I use it to make "white" breads, white crusty bread, the popular image of sourdough. Tempering the refined whiteness is the use of organic flour and the sourdough process, which avidly digests the flour, enhancing and converting it to a more suitable food than if the flour is used to make merely inflated (air-bag) bread.

There are many grades of "white" flour, some less sieved, even stone-ground first and then sieved. I'm using this type of flour for my "Casalinga" loaf at the time of writing. It is from South Australian medium-hard wheat. The creamy pale golden hue never ceases to please as I remove the dough after its first bulk proof.

Similarly the the stone-ground and then roller-milled, sieved biodynamic "white" bakers flour from Dayle Lloyd in south-west Western Australia, is tinged with a colour which can only be described as the hue of the magnificent "Salmon gums" which grace that area. It is truly arresting as one bakes with it regularly and is a benchmark flour.

It is worth looking for good flour like this, which reflects a "terroir" and is characteristic. "Terroir" is the best word to use as there is not really and English equivalent. "Terroir" is the whole of the influences of an area from topography to the seasons, every inherent factor which produces a noticeable character in food.

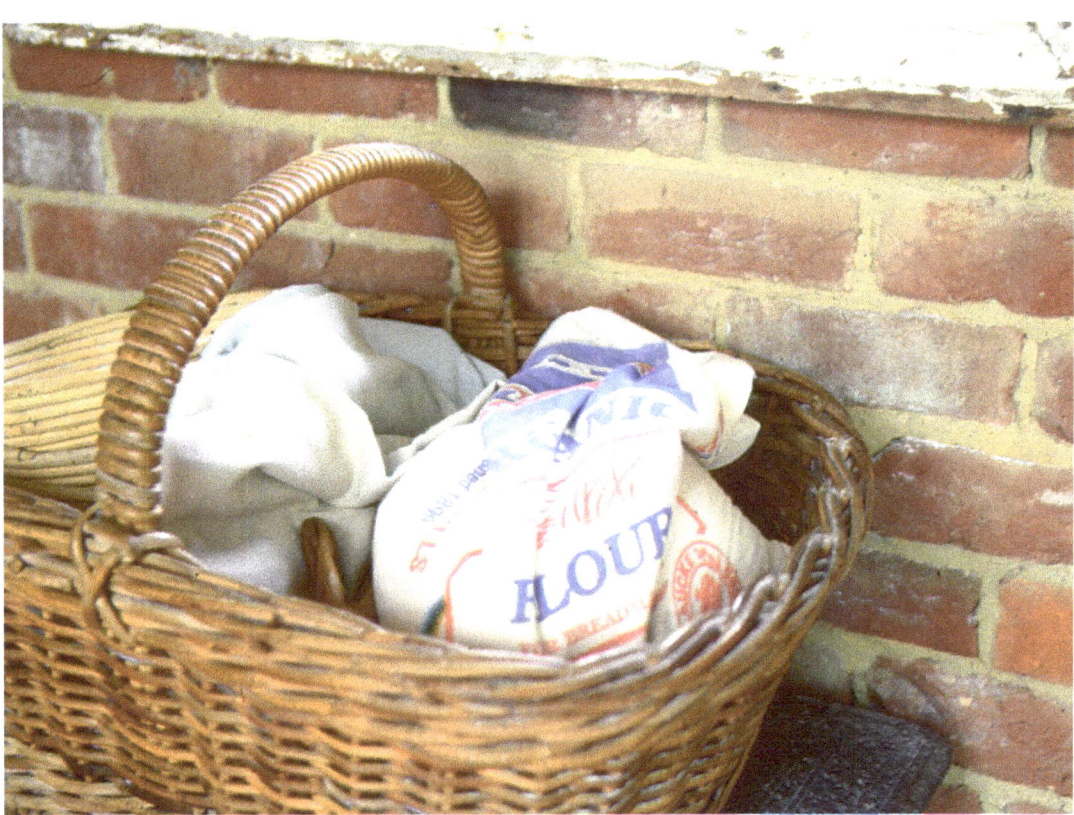

Most of you will seek the grail, which is the crusty white loaf. I usually temper white breads by using a leaven from wholemeal stoneground flour which has been sifted. Sifted stoneground flour is the most common flour used to make the classical and much adored traditional French bread - pain au levain. Indeed it is used in nearly all traditional bread, anywhere. The wholemeal flour is put in a mechanical sifter fitted with screens or sieves. This removes the very coarse particles of bran but retains the smaller particles of bran and germ. The essence of the bran and germ infuse the flour from the stone-grinding, so the flour is full-flavoured, yet lighter than a complete wholemeal.

This sifted-flour-leaven gives the white bread flavour which is usually missing in modern white bread, as the steel milling does not infuse white flour with the essence at all. Some millers call this sifted flour "light" or more horribly "lite", or 85% which means only 15% is removed as coarse bran. White flour is rated at approximately 70%, which means 30% is removed by refining.

Sifted flour is my choice and a traditional choice for everyday bread and gives the light golden-brown colour of those famous French loaves, the best crust and classical delicious wheaten flavour. It was also once used in the "Anglosphere" and the bread made from it was called "brown bread", as many bakeries had a mechanical flour sifter. Light flour can be made at home if you can acquire a fine sieve, simply run stoneground wholemeal through it a few times.

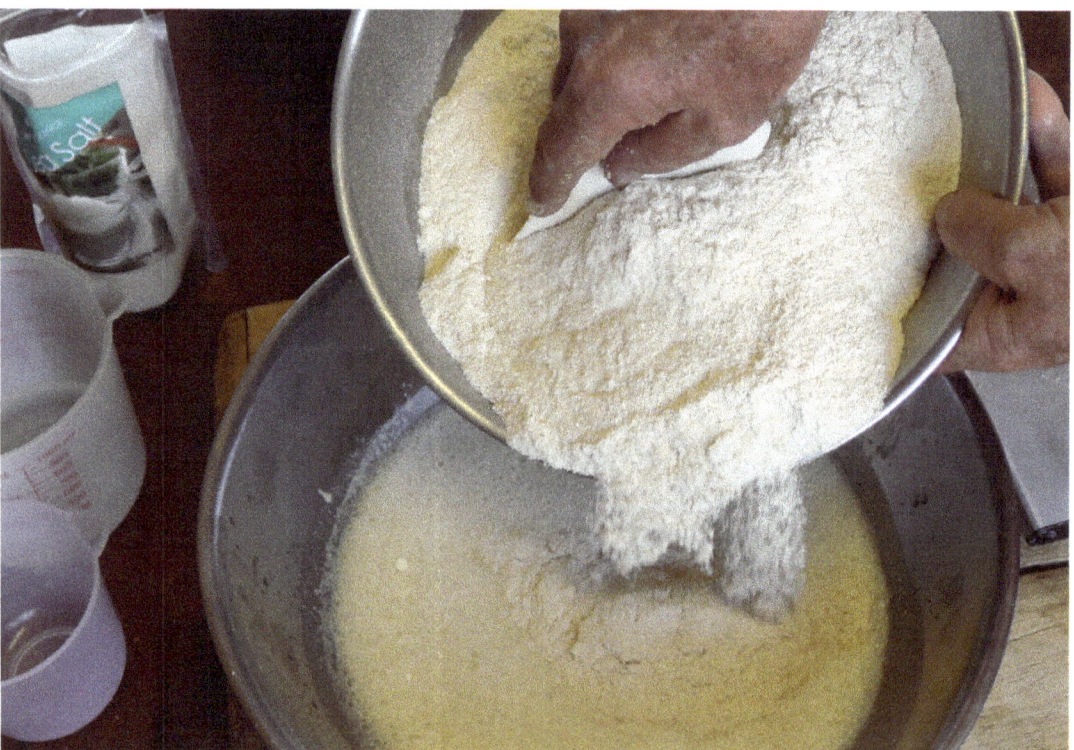

The Sourdough Loaf

Conventional wholemeal flour is made by firstly roller milling the wheat, sheering it into particles, sieving, and then re-combining the bran and germ with the white fraction. Part of my journey included worrying that my commercial leavens were not as active as I wanted or was used to, and realising I had started to use a roller-milled wholemeal which I conveniently ordered from the same mill as the white flour. Switching to stone-milled biodynamic wholemeal flour was eye-opening as after one week, my leavens were peaking and frothing again and producing more flavoursome bread.

In making bread you will have to use what you can source. The sourdough process itself often sorts out less than premium ingredients, and the results are always better than what can be generally purchased even-though they may not appear on the cover of a gourmet magazine. But how often have you purchased good-looking bread which failed to deliver the promise of the image?

Other Flours.

Flours other than wheat flour also vary considerably, meaning quantities aren't always exact. The rye of Europe is generally superior to Australian rye because Europeans use rye for bread, whereas the strains grown in Australia were mainly for stock feed. Rye contains very little gluten, the 'muscle' of wheat, and therefore high-rise is not an option in rye breads .

Nevertheless, good rye bread is relatively easy to make and rye flour can be blended with wheat flour to make "light" rye bread, famous as New York "deli" rye. Stoneground wholemeal rye always produces an active, easy to ferment leaven, and rye ferments easily to make good black bread which, while dense, digests easily and is full of flavour - and a brilliant hang-over cure!

Similarly, Spelt flour varies a lot and results vary widely depending on the type and origin of the spelt used. Spelt is in the wheat family, but as any baker knows, this doesn't mean much as it is less-forgiving than a good wheat bread-flour. Spelt does not have as much gluten as wheat yet it often has more protein, being the easily digested water soluble proteins which do not seem to upset the digestion of 'moderns' who have suffered from the western-pattern-diet - the WPD.

Spelt is usually available as a wholemeal or as "white" , which appears very white until water is added and its dun-hue is revealed. It is not roller-milled usually, but a sifted, stone ground flour.

Spelt makes very good bread if handled carefully and similar to rye, produces very active leavens. Some types of Spelt can give a magnificent "shaley" crust, especially in baguette or crusty hearth breads. Fanatics will want to make authentic baguette using sifted spelt flour with a short ferment of soft dough and a hot oven, another panary benchmark.

Varieties of Wheat Flours.

Other varieties of wheat are now commonly available which also make good bread and appear not to be as allergenic as modern wheat can be to some. Commonly, Kamut is available but this is a trademark name for a variety of durum wheat sourced from an Egyptian farmer and brought to the USA after World War II.

The correct name for this wheat is Khorassan and it is widely used in India, Iran, Pakistan and Egypt. One miller has called it "Egyptian gold". Khorassan has great flavour and makes excellent flat or flatter breads as are widely made in the countries mentioned, notably the primal bread from a wood-fired tandoor oven, often called Naan.

Khorassan does not have the gluten content of regular bread wheat and again appears to be less allergenic to those made wheat-sensitive by the WPD. It makes well-flavoured structured bread with sensitive handling. Khorassan can also be mixed with regular wheat flour for enhanced flavour and similarly can be sifted although when stoneground it tends to be more gritty with less flaky bran, so more of the grain will go through the sifter.

We are now fortunate to have access to more ancient, less hybridised members of the wheat family, carrying tastes from vanished centuries, which again appear to be less allergenic to those sensitive.

I have been using Emmer wheat for some time and find it to be superbly flavoured. Emmer is almost the oldest wheat variety and was the staple of ancient Egypt and Rome. It was surprising to find emmer (farro) widely available in Italian stores/supermarkets but it has always been a remnant crop since Roman times - tangible history.

Emmer makes the best flatbreads with full flavour and a dense chewy texture. Also a brilliant (the best) pizza base, common in central and northern Italy. The original focaccia was so made, a far cry from the white slab now sold under this name. Emmer is widely available although pricey as the yield is much lower than modern wheat, so farmers demand a higher price.

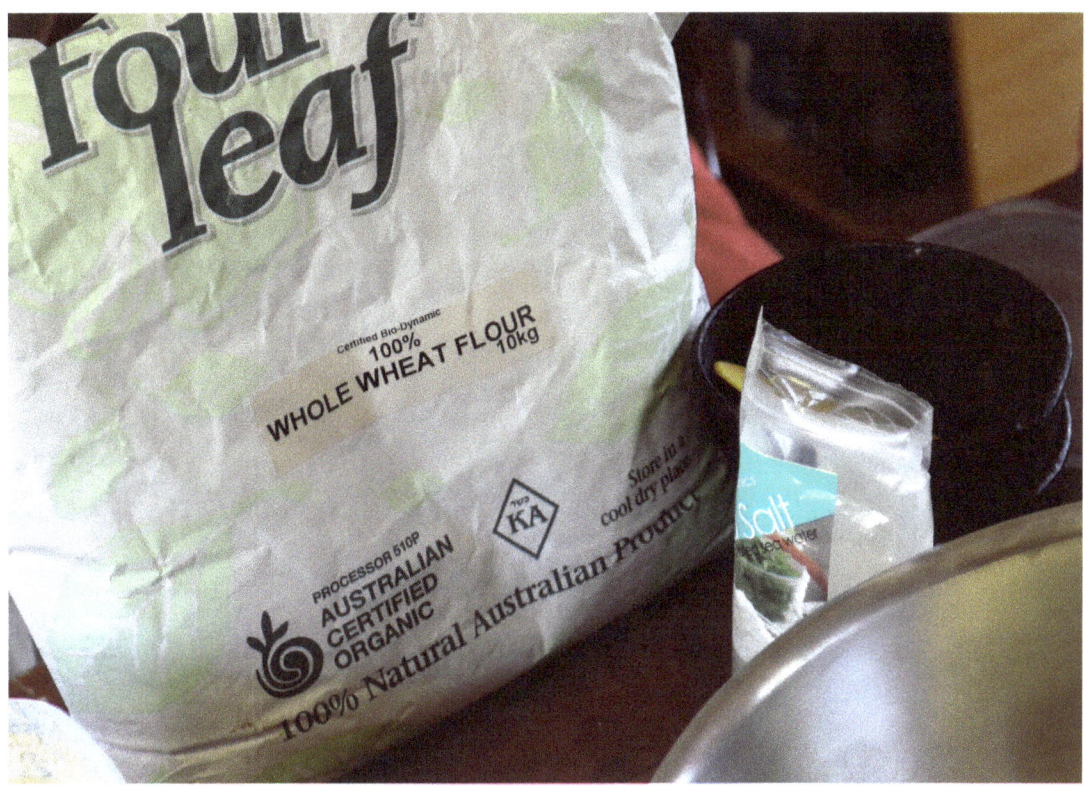

The very oldest wheat is also becoming available and this is Einkorn. This grain has a distinct flavour, or complex "progenitor" flavour as it embodies the taste of "cereal" - earthy, nutty and farinaceous. It is a very soft wheat, having much lower gluten content but higher protein than modern wheat, these being again the water-soluble proteins.

It is not easy to get good bread structure with einkorn, although it can be done with skill, so it is most suitable for making delicious flat breads or mixing with stronger flours for added flavour. Einkorn will vary depending on where it was grown and how it was milled, and it does make the very best biscuits.

Heritage Wheat.

Recently while working in the UK I was privileged to make bread from heritage wheat strains grown by John Letts who assiduously collected these strains from seed banks and obscure locations. Andrew Forbes has also collected some of the original strains which were once prized in the UK for full-flavoured bread, well-adapted to local climate or terroir.

These heritage wheat strains, far from being simply groovy or for the "rarity obsessed" are important culturally, historically and genetically. They also make benchmark-tasty bread, which is why they were originally selected and grown for hundreds of years. With industrialisation, flavour was superseded by yield, convenience of mechanical harvesting and broad-scale farming.

It has seemingly been forgotten that bread is food, the most common food, and for many, the staple. Heritage wheats remind us of a quality and meaning now largely forgotten, combining enhanced nutrition through low gluten and more protein than modern wheat, with wonderfully satisfying flavour and bloomy colour fused with ancestral emotion.

I was truly surprised by the flavour of heritage wheat, although I had glimpsed it in Australia from the almost-heritage falcon wheat variety, grown until recently, and now revived by biodynamic farmers at Eden valley in Western Australia as a part of their grist. It was the first good flour I had as a struggling commercial baker trying to source anything but the very ordinary available flours.

The English heritage wheat had been stoneground and was a wholemeal. The bread which resulted was dense yet light to eat. The crumb was more like a delicate cake redolent of lost flavours of wheaten goodness. The crust was burnished and cacao-like, with layers of flavour from roasted chestnuts and chicory; a true gastronomic experience yet humble and earthy, another tangible and timeless link.

If you can get access to these flours, which are available in the UK, France and the USA (and possibly online elsewhere), do try them to experience the sort of flavour and texture and yes, romance, missing in today's prosaic panary.

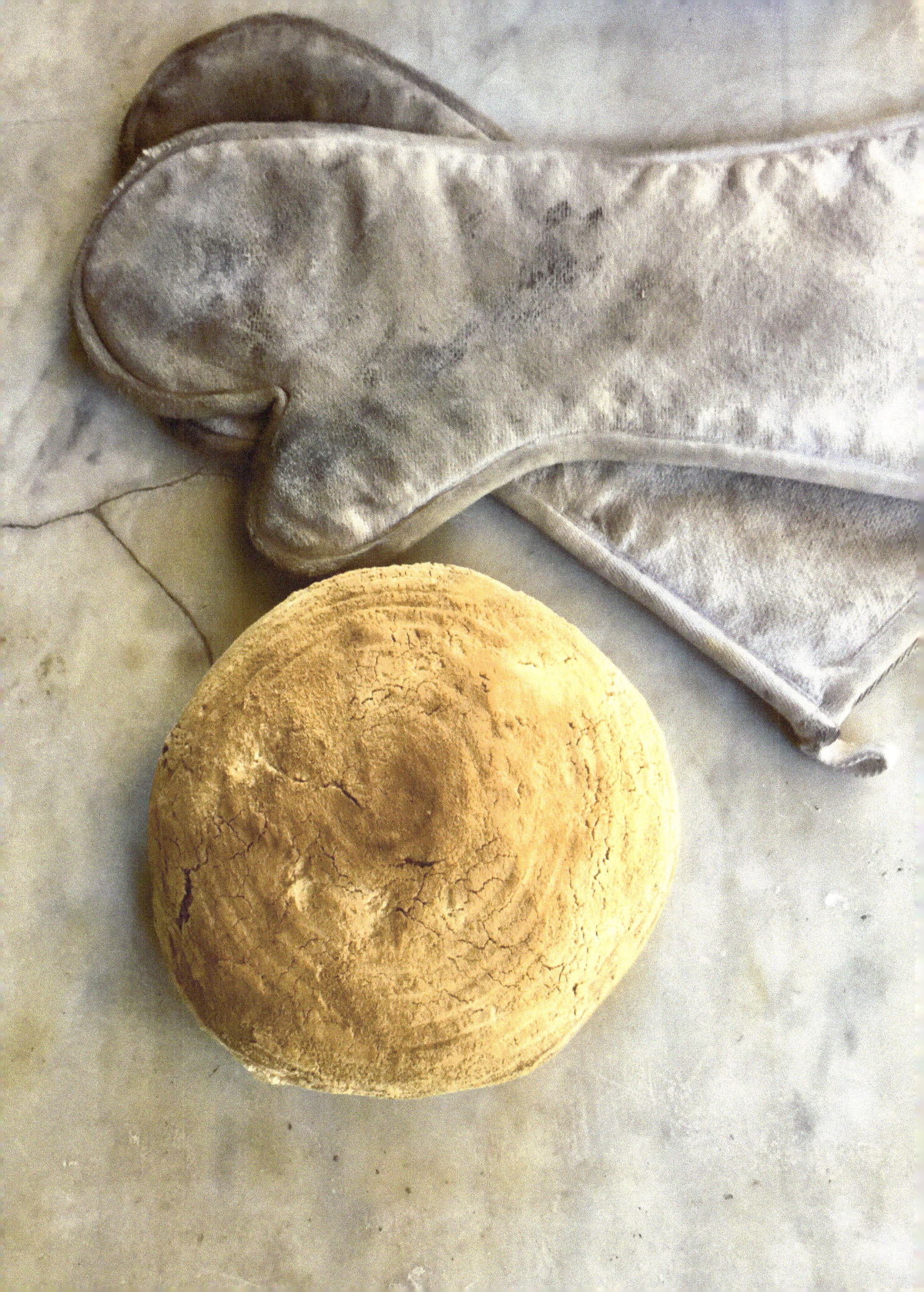

STAIRWAY TO LEAVEN
How to start and manage a relationship.

A friend once called sourdough bread "The philosopher's stone" and there is truth in this, as the sourdough process transforms hard and flinty grain into a flavoursome, digestible, nutritious treasure. The real "secret" is in the growth and maintenance of the starter/culture, historically called, the leaven. This is the key to unlocking the treasure.

Be prepared. It may overtake your life as partner/family/pets will all desert you as the obsession grows. However they will eventually return just to eat your delicious bread.

The role of the leaven.

To make a sourdough bread, the sourdough leaven is mixed with more flour, water and salt to make a dough, which will ferment and rise, and is then baked. The leaven simply replaces the addition of yeast; the sourdough will rise more slowly but the process is essentially the same, although the result is very different.

This recipe aims to produce a 500g sourdough leaven for use in home baking. You may wish to adjust the quantities to make more or less to suit your needs, but if you stick to the relative proportions used here, there should be no problems.

I don't claim this to be the only way to initiate a leaven as there are other ways, but this is what I have always done and it works.

Ingredients:

- *125g organic or biodynamic, stoneground wholemeal wheat flour.*
- *190g slightly warm water.*

Use a bowl for the mixing and the initiation. Later, when the leaven becomes active, transfer to a suitable permanent home. I always used a glass jar until it was dropped one day. Since then my leaven has happily lived in a plastic tub, once containing honey.

Initiation.

Day 1

Mix the ingredients well and cover with a cotton tea-towel and place in a draught-free, "not cold" spot. Leave undisturbed overnight or for about 12 hours.

Day 2

Give the mix a good stir and replace the tea-towel.

Choose a time which is convenient and try to attend to the leaven at a similar time each day if possible. This is initially important, but will be less demanding as the leaven becomes established.

Days 3-6

Check the leaven and stir it each day, and when there are little bubbles, things are moving. The arcane reference is that "the angels of air" have entered the culture. As the activity progresses, more bubbles, and a pleasant sourish, yeasty, grassy aroma is evident. The leaven is on the way and time to move to the next stage, which is growth.

If your leaven is not on the way, stir and walk away until the next day. Activity is more likely to be evident in summer, but in cold climates, be patient. If no activity has happened by day 5, it is a concern, persevere for another day but you may have to start again.

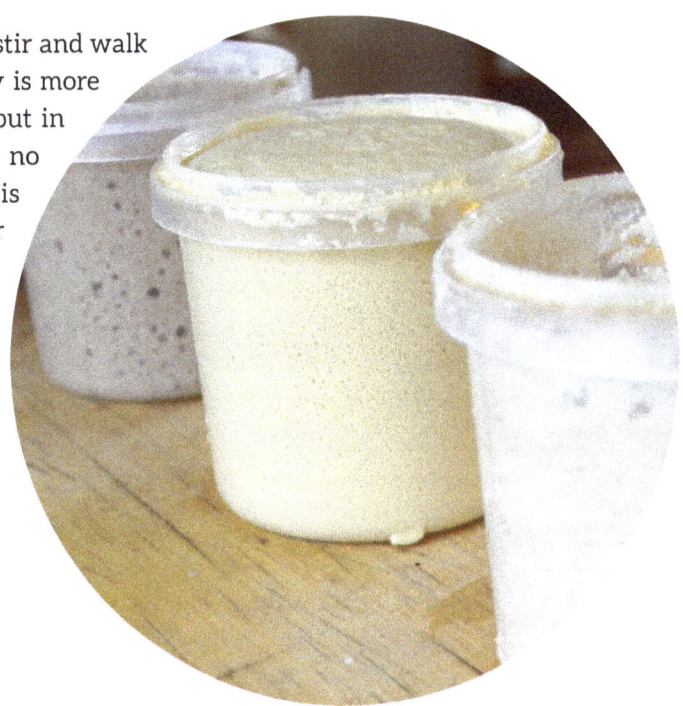

Growth.

Day 1.

The leaven should now be clearly active, hopefully frothing and bubbling. Celebrate the arrival of your new life partner!.

Add to the newly active culture, the original ingredients:
125g wholemeal flour and 190g water.

Stir these in to make a smooth thick batter.

Days 2 - 4.

Pour off half of the leaven, and refresh the remnant half with the original quantities of flour and water and stir once again to make a smooth batter. Continue this refreshment each day for 3 days until the leaven is well established.
The discarded portion can be mixed with flour and water/milk to make crackers or pancakes for your first taste (refer to "Bread of the Rings" in the recipes section), or compost it.

After 3 days the leaven should be clearly active, frothing and bubbling, rising in the container with a pleasant sourish aroma and ready for bread-making.

The leaven will rise up and be active for hours after feeding. Once it has peaked, it will settle and remain dormant for some time until "fed" again. It should be used at the peak.

Storing and refreshing the leaven.

Each time the leaven is used to make bread, be sure to reserve at least 2 tablespoons in order to seed the next batch. Add the same amount of flour (125g) and water (190g) (or those ratios if making larger quantities) to the reserved seed leaven and stir in well. It should be ready for baking in about 8 hours.

If you aren't baking with it daily, you can refrigerate it. An active starter can be refrigerated for quite some time, but to remain functional, it needs to be refreshed weekly. After a week of refrigeration, remove from the fridge and allow it to return to room temperature. It can then be refreshed by pouring off half and adding the original amount of flour and water, and returning it to the fridge.

Preparation for Breadmaking.

If you want to make bread from the refrigerated leaven, simply add the original amount of flour and water and leave it out of the fridge to re-activate, usually 8 hours. It is then ready for bread-making. A shortcut is to simply stir a few tablespoons of flour into the leaven when it is just out of the fridge to form a very thick batter, which will activate it more quickly.

As a commercial baker and fanatic, I never refrigerate the leaven. This ensures a rapid response and ensures that it is highly active. If you bake regularly I recommend not refrigerating it, but refreshing daily, always discarding half, which can be composted or used for ring breads. Refreshing every second, even third day is fine in cool weather. Otherwise, refrigerate. It will work well but may be slightly sleepy and a little slower.

Trick of the trade.

When the leaven peaks, rising up in the container and is strongly active, stir it well using a wooden spoon. This reduces its volume, but the fermentation is stimulated and re-activates quickly, becoming more liquid and rising again.

Bakers call this "knocking back" and its function is to potentiate the ferment. It should be peaking again after 3 hours and must be used then or the leaven lapses and becomes dormant. This is not an essential step, but definitely primes the leaven and makes better bread.

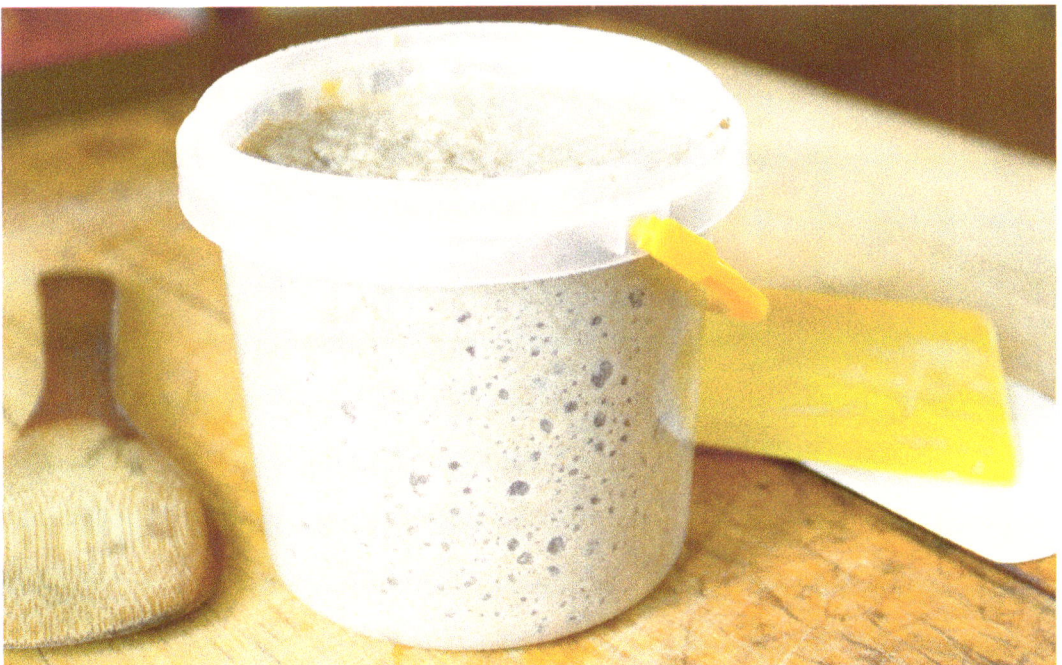

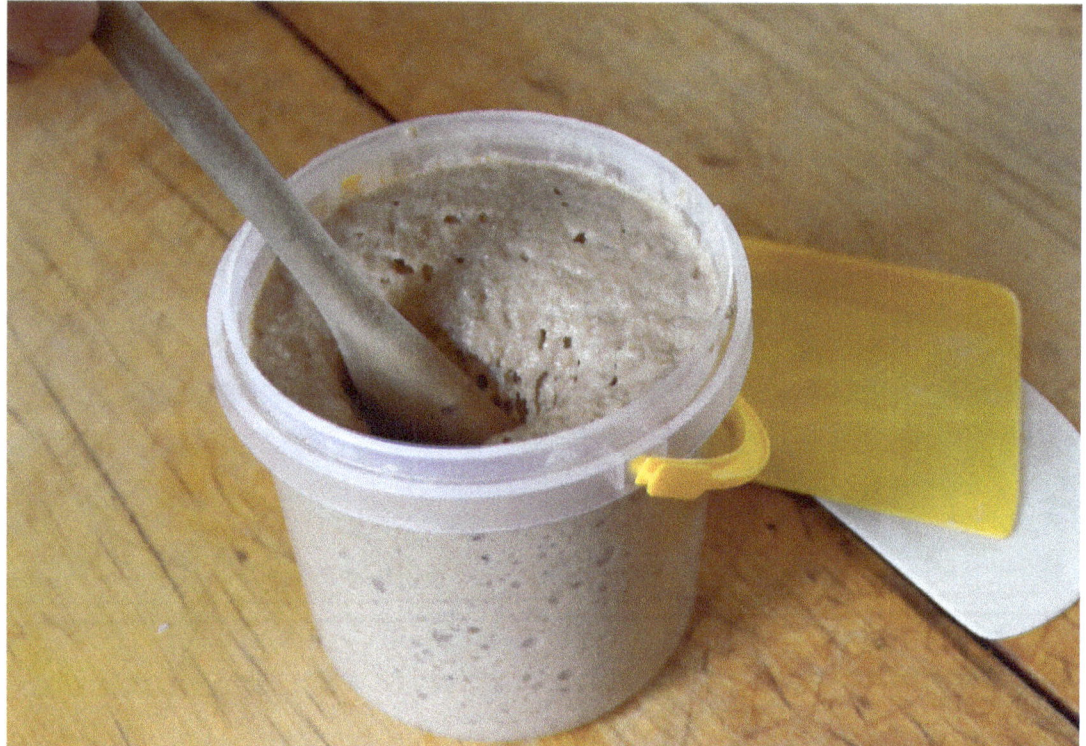

Consistency.

The newly-made leaven should have the consistency of a very thick batter. This will thin down as it ferments, and be more liquid by the time it is ready to use. Starting with a too-thin leaven will lead to increased sourness and less rising power.

Water.

It is ideal to use spring water, but costly. Even more ideal is to use rainwater. It is true that a poor ferment can be caused by unsuitable water, or killed outright. This process works with tap water and I always use tap water. Trouble-shooting must include different water if the process is not working.

Flour.

The regular leaven needs to be made from organic, or bio-dynamic, stoneground wholemeal wheat flour. Using this flour will ensure success. Maintaining a white-flour leaven is not as satisfactory in flavour or activity. The microbiome in a wholegrain matrix is far more complex and the organisms are more robust. This regular wholemeal leaven is called the "stock" or "seed" leaven.

The wholemeal leaven makes a really good "white" bread when used with white flour, but for a whiter loaf, make a white leaven from the stock. Make the original leaven quantities with white flour and stir in 2 tablespoons of the wholemeal stock. A white leaven takes longer to ripen than a wholemeal, an hour or two extra, so make sure to give it time. This will also need to be stirred well when it peaks and allowed to re-activate for a few hours before use.

Using sifted wholemeal, "light" flour makes the most outstanding leaven for white bread. The loaf is very lightly coloured but the flavour from the brown leaven is exceptional and the crust is well-coloured and well developed. To make the brown leaven, simply use the original leaven quantities using sifted wholemeal and stir in 2 tablespoons of the wholemeal stock.

New leavens can be created in this way. For example cacao powder used instead of flour and seeded with the stock makes a powerful and exotic leaven to be used in a very special bread. Bread containing cacao was common once. Similarly rye or brown rice flour or sorghum flour can be used for a leaven instead of wheat flour to make gluten-free products. These can be seeded with the wheat leaven stock initially and then once established, regularly refreshed with gluten-free grain flour.

If you aren't having success initiating a leaven from scratch, begin troubleshooting by trying different flour. In my experience, stone-ground wholemeal wheat flour makes the best leaven, but this does not mean it cannot be done with other flour. Sometimes, using rye or spelt flour will initiate the leaven more easily and is well worth trying if you aren't having success. Simply follow the leaven-making instructions using wholemeal rye or spelt flour.

Temperature.

Ambient "room" temperature of course varies with climate. In Australia at 40°C, the leaven will go "off" in 12 hours, which means it sours rapidly, so the refreshment schedule needs to be adjusted if you do not refrigerate the leaven. A friend in Spain told me he refreshes 2-3 times a day in 40 degree weather - perhaps a case for refrigeration! During an English winter a warmish spot is needed or something like an electric blanket. The ideal temperature is about 25 degrees. Be vigilant and observe the cycle of your starter, act accordingly, and this attention initiates good bread.

Smells.

If you have tried and have a really unpleasant smell after a few days, throw it away and start again. Believe me it is not worth persevering with a smelly leaven, although some do. Next time, perhaps clean the receptacle with boiling water, wash everything and make sure all the implements are very clean. If the leaven spot is too warm/hot a bad fermentation can easily result.

Leaven.

What you have made is variously called "the starter", "the culture" or "the leaven". Leaven is certainly the time-honoured term, known as "le levain" (m) in French. Technically and grammatically, it is not a "mother".

Leaven: Ultimatum.

The leaven is absolutely important to all, so if you have not been successful in your attempts to make a leaven as directed, beg, borrow or steal one. Find someone who has a good leaven and hopefully they will give you some. Alternatively, marry somebody who has one, which in the before time, was considered a good reason. Leavens are available online, dried and fresh, and in this way, get some, prove your love and the leaven will be yours as long as the love is there.

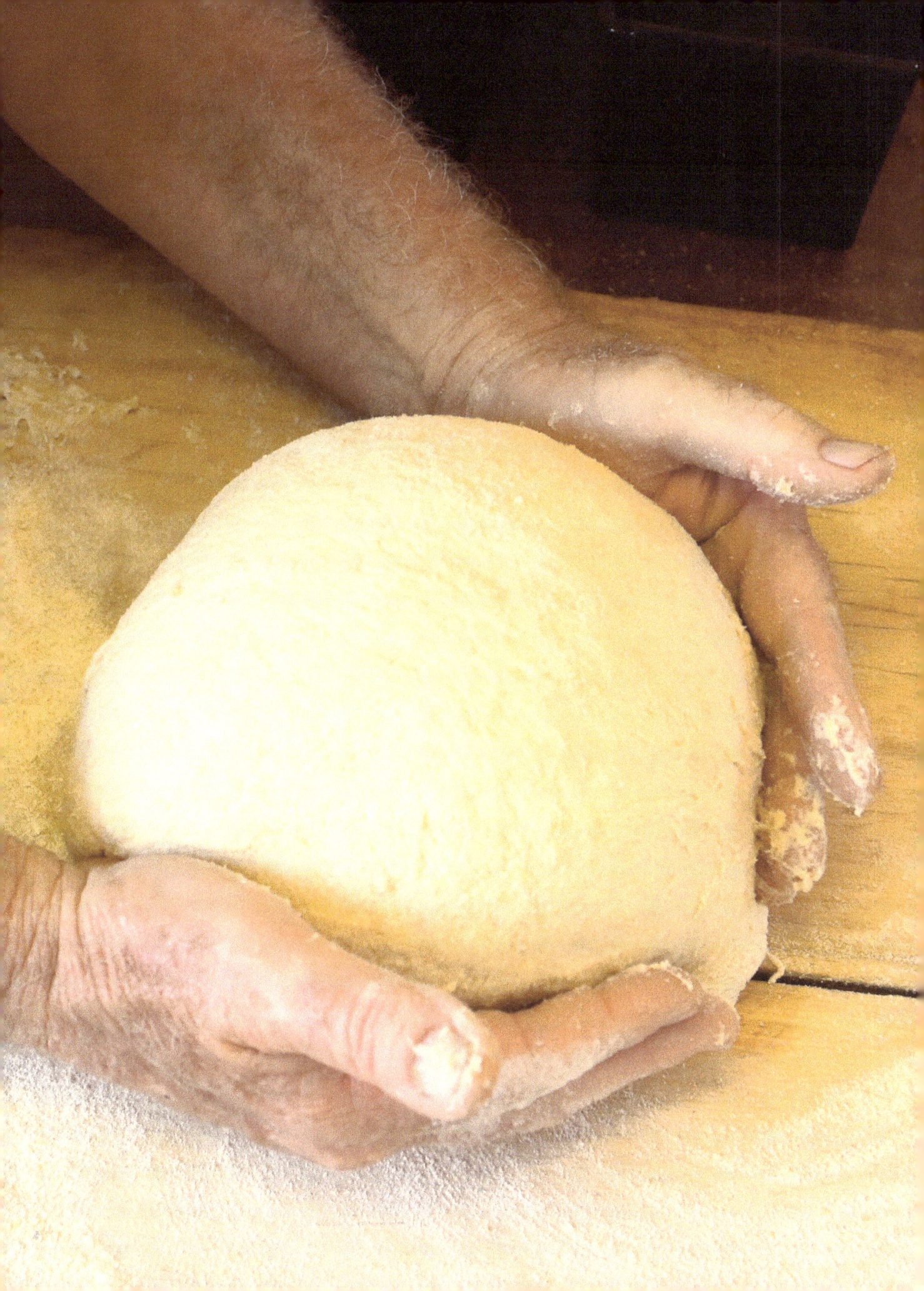

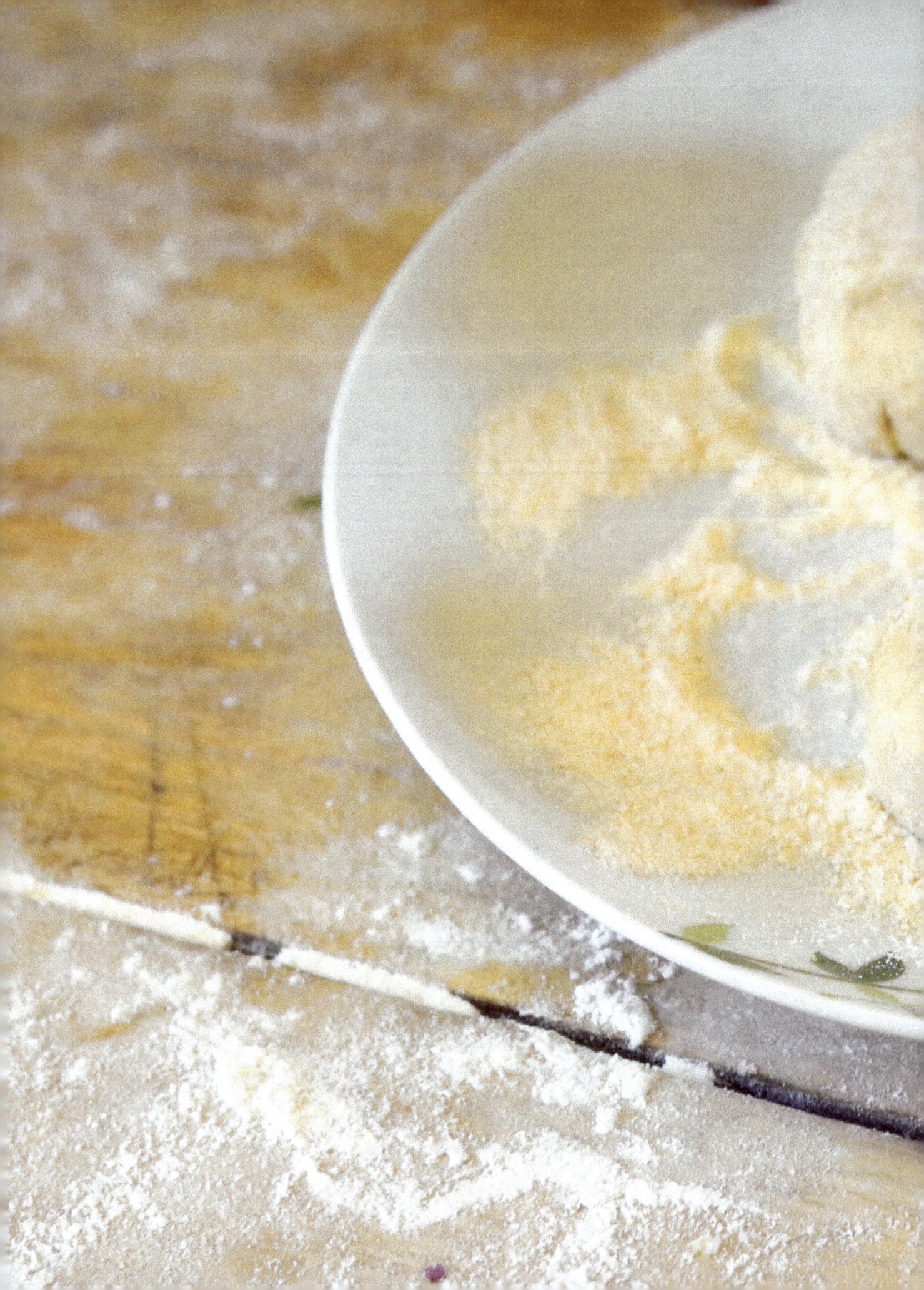

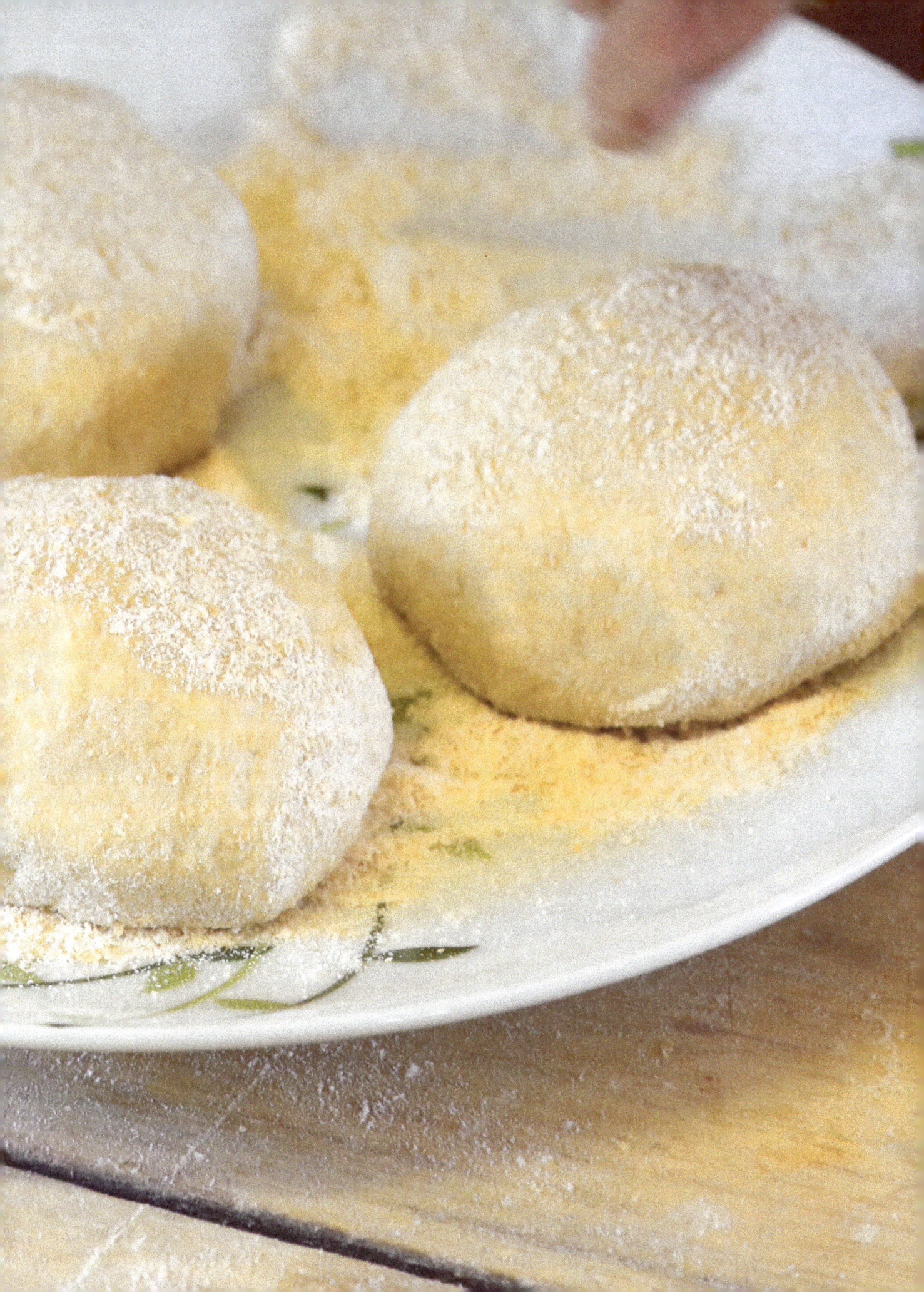

DAD'S WHEAT

It was a chance meeting, a shared hotel, both overnighting from the country, both facing bad news at the hospital tomorrow. We passed, pacing distractedly and met, staring out over the city, too late at night.

He was in his 70s, I was 48. We talked about anything but why we were there. Bread came up. Like lots of "old-timers", imprinted experiences flowed freely. The best bit for me was his story about his Dad's wheat.

His father always grew what he called "an old variety" of wheat which he thought had come with his father's father from the old country. He said it was very tall, "taller than a man" and he always received a premium price from the millers.

But most notable when, due to poor seasons or pestilence, other crops failed, his father's always produced well. He laughed and shot off that all the other farmers who'd usually got their wheat seed from the "gubberment" "Ag" department, came and got seed from him, and he was happy to supply it.

These naturally bred and selected, ideal bread wheats have all but disappeared, although some are now attracting major attention among sustainable-agriculture farmers, and bakers with soul.

Barley.

Less common bread-making flours were once widely used, usually without wheat flour, which was scare or unknown in many areas. Barley was widely used to make bread in Europe and Asia, also being the commonest flour in the British Isles.

Barley was usually made into a flatbread called bannock in Scotland, but made throughout the "Celtic" world, baked in the ashes or on a griddle. It was usually fully fermented, or left to "turn" for a while, providing aeration, digestibility and new flavour. Barley and oats were also used to make extremely delicious sourdough "cakes" and crumpet-like items in the north of England, Scotland and Eire which are demonstrated in the recipe section titled "Bread of the Rings". These were usually made from a fine meal.

Barley is still widely used in the Himalayas, notably Tibet, where it is lightly roasted to accentuate flavour. It can be added to any of the breads here as a quarter to a third of the total flour quantity. Using more is tricky unless one is used to it, as the bread tends to be quite dense. The best way to use barley or oats in regular bread, is to make the leaven from these grains and then add regular flour. This really brings out the flavour and aroma of the grains.

They can also be made into a thick porridge and mixed in to the dough, for a flavoursome dense crumb, similar to the corn bread described below.

Millet.

I was fortunate to be ushered into an Ethiopian kitchen in London to watch the sourdough millet flatbread *injera* being made. Injera is made from a type of millet called Teff traditionally, but usually has a proportion of wheat flour added outside Ethiopia today. Injera is spongey, lacey, unusually coloured and very sour with a bitter edge. Accompanying it are fiery vegetable, meat and legume dishes. All challenging flavours.

Teff is expensive outside Ethiopia where it is a staple, but finely ground yellow millet flour is widely available in the west and can be used as a substitute, but again, it is strongly flavoured. The ideal way to use millet flour is to toast it gently first. It can be added to most bread recipes, at no more than 10% of the total flour weight. Millet can also be used as is Chickpea flour in the Soca recipe.

Corn.

Corn bread was a very successful loaf in my early bakery and is indeed tasty and attractively coloured. I used yellow polenta for this loaf. The polenta is first cooked or soaked in boiling water to soften its flinty texture and draw out the pleasing flavour of corn/maize. This step is

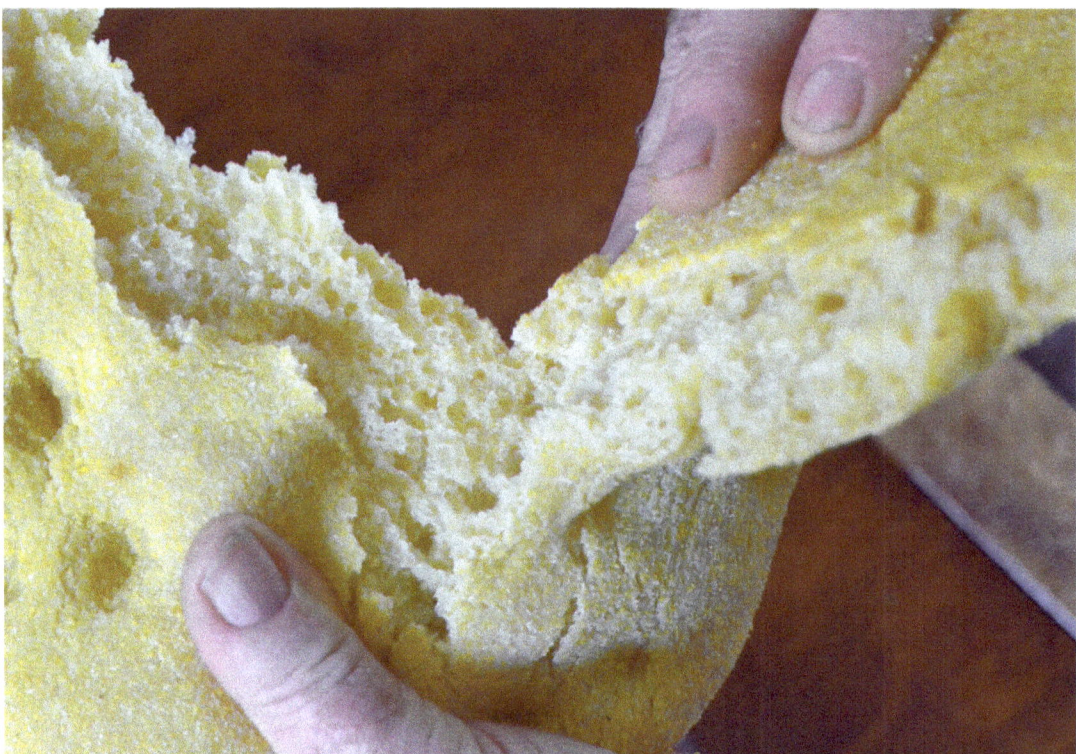

necessary otherwise the dry meal draws moisture from the loaf and the texture becomes hard.

Corn/maize meal can be replaced with masa harina which is a corn flour which has been nixtamalised (soaked in wood-ash solution, lye) to correct its tendency to bind B vitamins.

Other grains.

There are other flours to experiment with such as chestnut flour, chickpea flour (besan), brown rice or quinoa flour. Chestnut flour makes a superb leaven which can then be mixed with wheat flour to make earthy flatbreads with rustic and appealing semi-sweet flavour.

Explore the Soca, chickpea flatbread recipe which is one of the oldest flatbreads. More of a pancake or pan-bread, this salty spicey bread was once common on the Mediterranean rim and harks from ancient Punic and Roman roots. It also resembles South Indian Dosa in technique.

The technique for making Soca is an education in using non-wheat flours and moving outside the envelope of risen European type breads. It is an ideal path to making gluten-free breads rather than bothering to make risen gluten-free "breads" using cumbersome artifice and strange ingredients.

These flatbreads are arcane, nourishing and exciting from a gastronomic angle. They can be filled and rolled up, torn and eaten with the hands, dipped into or enrobing other foods for casual dining.

A common example of gluten-free traditional bread is the buckwheat crepe of Brittany. This batter is left to ferment before being spread on a hotplate to cook or poured into a waffle iron for effect. The lacey texture is easy to achieve if the batter is left to "turn", the old expression, and nicely accompanies other food with its earthy flavour. Buckwheat flour is widely available and well worth trying. The batter can be left in the refrigerator and used to make appetising "fast food" sourdough crepes, pancakes or waffles accompanied by good cheese and green leaves, a brilliant quick meal.

> *Grind the grain by hand*
>
> *Add rainwater and coloured salt*
>
> *The angels of air will enter and grow within*
>
> *Bake with fire.*

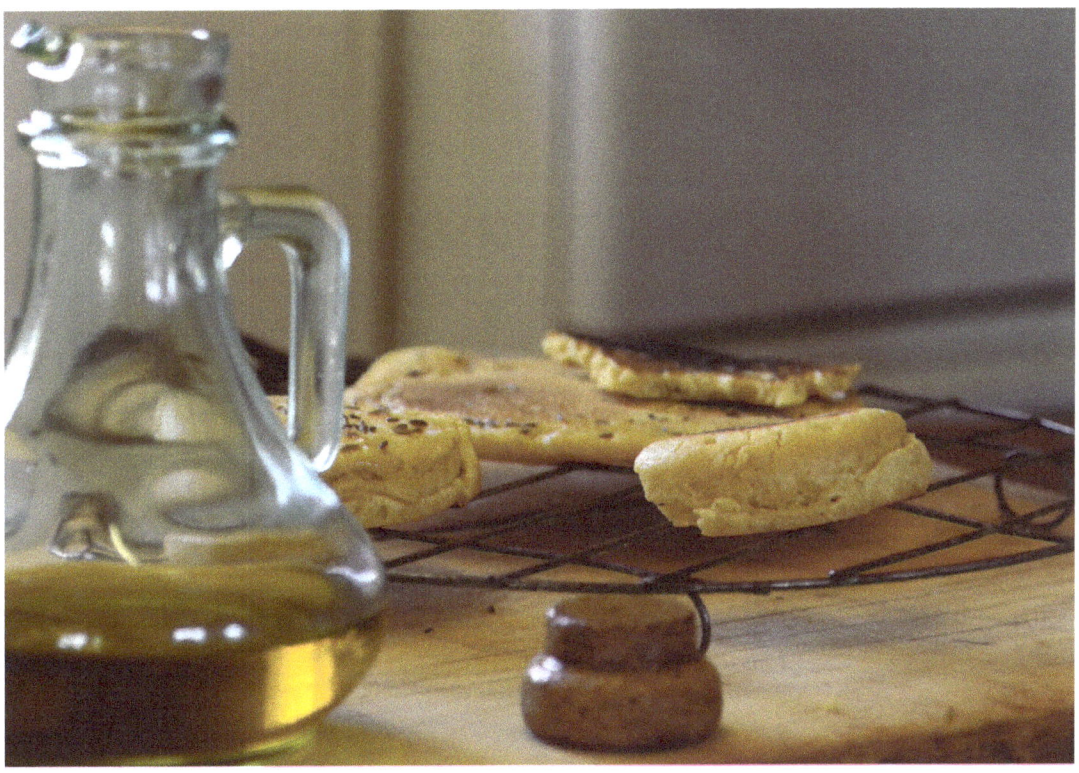

Water.

Old-time bakers swore that rainwater made the best bread. Clearly the quality of water is important in bread making, but not enough for most to bother with. Tap water is generally suitable. Good water does help in the subtle quality of the bread and those with rural rainwater are fortunate as there is a nice cosmic synergy with grain and rainwater - and I'm sure there are scientific factoids as well.

> *Leave out a bowl*
>
> *Collect rainwater*
>
> *Make bread.*

Salt.

The third part of the three jewels of bread-making is Salt.

There is no doubt that the grey salt collected in the traditional way by sun-drying, basically evaporating the seawater, contains trace elements which enable all sorts of biological pathways. Regular salt is simply sodium chloride, two elements, and nearly always today is contaminated with "anti-caking" agents. Iodised salt is now common. Himalayan pink and salt from the mountains of the moon are available....these all perform the same astringent function and create balance. Best practice is to purchase salt which is additive-free.

Enhanced nutrition and primordial salinity comes from the grey or coloured salt. It has significant tang when used on top of flatbreads, really enhancing flavour and promoting the experience.

Traditionally, salt was valued for enabling bread and cereals to be more digestible.

> *Collect the foaming surf.*
>
> *Build a fire on the beach.*
>
> *Make salt.*

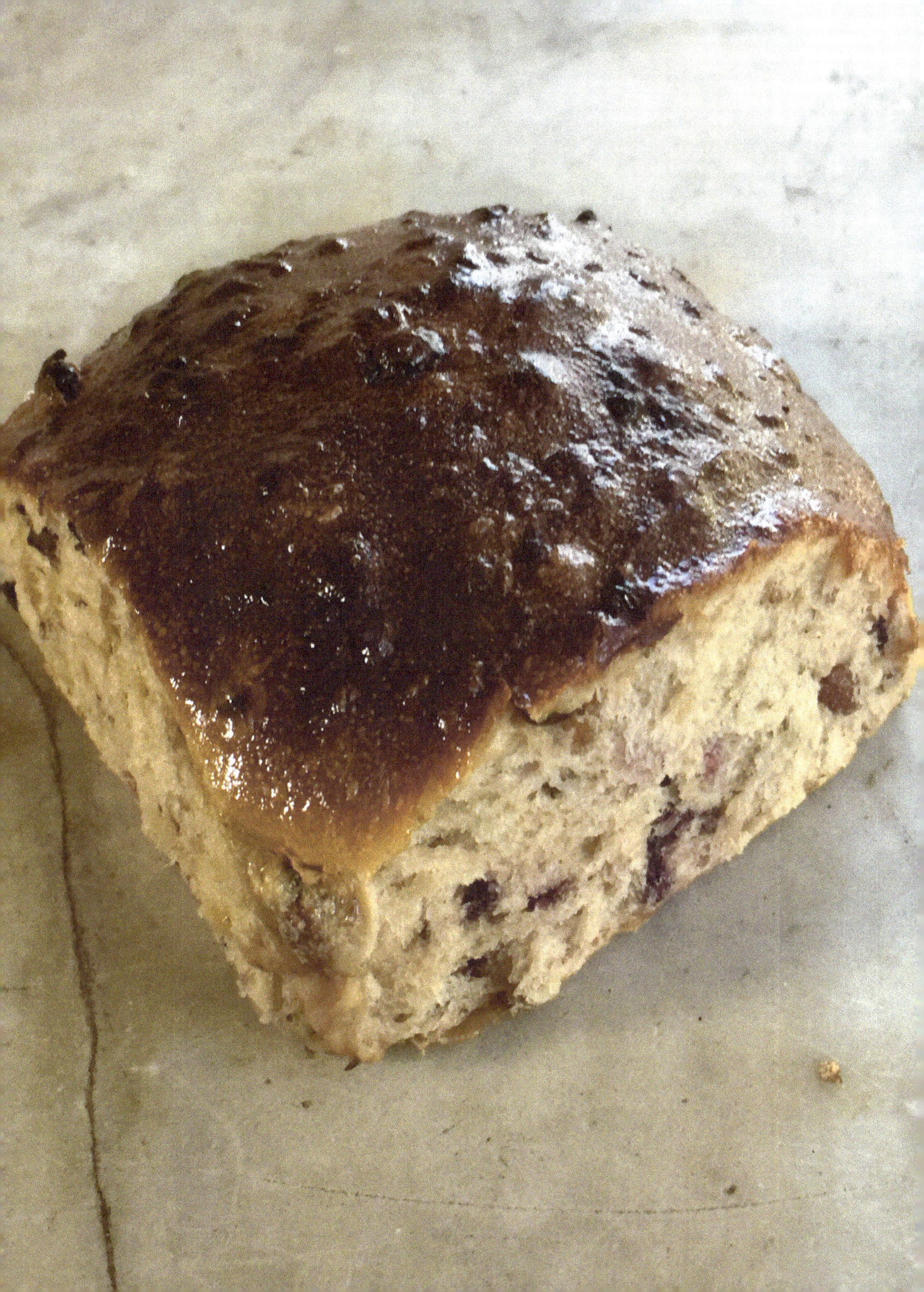

EQUIPMENT FOR BAKING.

Most of us are familiar with the rectangular-cuboid loaf, perhaps with a domed top, which is baked in a metal tin. This tin is a relatively recent tool in bread baking.

Those familiar with sourdough bread will mostly have purchased it or will have noticed the less-mechanical free-form or crusty shape, a round or torpedo shape with cuts or slashes in the crust, often bursting with colour, artistry and aesthetic appeal.

This does not mean sourdough cannot be baked in a tin, and often the tinned shape is considered more convenient. Crust lovers usually don't even notice tinned breads, and in Melbourne, my European customers actually disdained them. Convenience lovers, however, feel the crusty shape "doesn't fit in the toaster". Both the crusty loaf and the tin loaf are explored in the recipe section.

Besides a basket or tin, the leaven and the flour, it is important to have on hand a few easily accessed tools at bread-baking time.

A good-sized stainless steel or pottery bowl.

This should be big enough to mix, knead and play around in as you develop the correct texture. A bowl with diameter of 37cm is ideal. If the bowl is much smaller, dramas will befall you. This sized bowl can contain 2kg of dough comfortably, which is probably more than usually required, but leaves plenty of elbow-room for mixing and rising.

At home I mix the dough in this bowl, remove it to a suitable flat surface for some kneading, which isn't absolutely necessary if you are kneading-challenged, and then put the dough back in the bowl for rising, which bakers call "proof" or "proving". It needs to be a "friendly" bowl. A smaller bowl for use on scales and dissolving salt should also be a part of the bread kit.

A good strong wooden spoon for mixing.

Metal spoons can be used but wooden spoons have a certain appeal which is more conducive to this process. Ensure the spoons are stout as a thin handle will easily snap.

Scales.

These are essential for weighing flour, water, salt and other ingredients.

A baker's "slip".

This is a small thin plastic spatula-like half-disc which is indispensable - the baker's third hand. The slip can slide under doughs, mix, scoop-up, and incorporate ingredients with ease, and alleviate sticky-dough-on-the-hands syndrome. Some call it a "scraper"!

A Whisk.

Largely for whisking mixes of water and leaven. This aerates the leaven-water mix, promoting activity and a sweeter dough.

A Scoop.

A scoop or favourite cup/small bowl for adding flour or other ingredients.

Tea towels.

A few good thick cotton tea-towels, ideally kept for bread making only. These cover rising doughs and dry tears of elation or despair at your efforts.

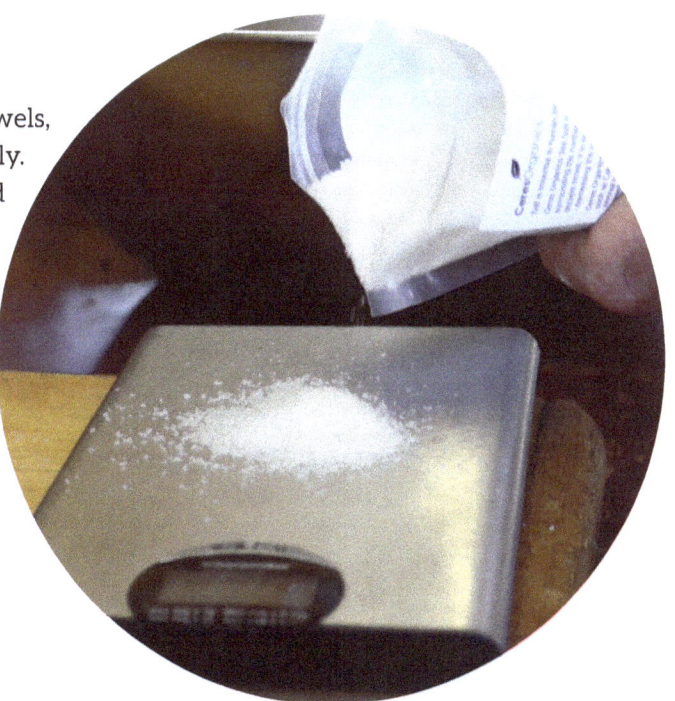

A plastic bag.

Good-sized plastic bags such as kitchen-tidy bags. I know, plastic, but unless you can

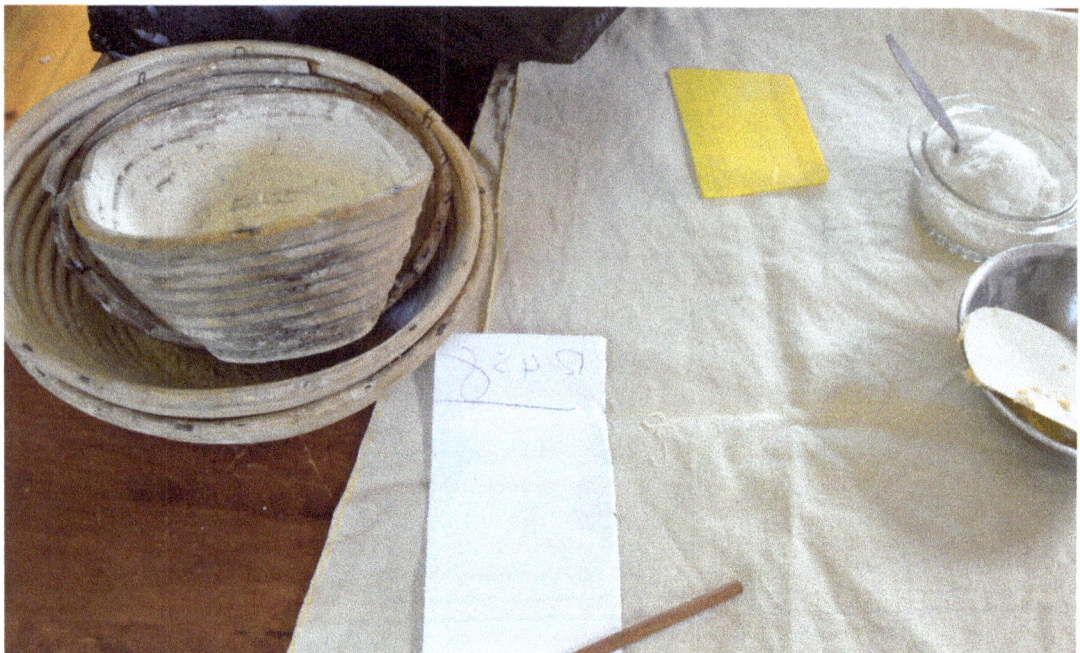

source oiled-cloth or vellum from the luddite store, plastic bags are perfect for maintaining dough moisture. They also prevent the formation of a "skin" on the dough which may spoil the texture and prevent a good rise. The same bag can be reused many times.

Bread tins.

An ideal loaf tin is 25cm long, 10cm high, 12cm wide at the top and 9cm wide at the base. These do vary, but that approximate size is most suitable, suiting two loaves of panes cum toto for example. Smaller tins are useful but larger are problematic in that the larger amount of dough they contain takes longer to bake and the heat of a domestic oven may not penetrate to the centre of the loaf ... which is heart-breaking if the rest of the loaf is nicely baked but the centre is raw-ish.

Banneton or baskets.

Banneton are baskets made of cane specifically for rising a crusty loaf. They can be purchased as oblong-torpedo shapes, large and small, or as rounds. The banneton is to be well-floured and the dough is placed in it for its final, pre-oven rise. The torpedo shape is practical and what I used for my original "Casalinga" loaf, now popular in Melbourne, and instantly recognisable as a sourdough.

I really like the round loaf shape but this is not as popular commercially, largely because, again, "it doesn't fit in the toaster", and the irregular slices aren't suitable for wrapped lunches. Further, there is always a crust leftover…the small remnant end-piece which used to be given to "swaggies" in the before time.

There is an ancestral appeal, even an ancestral emotion, about the round loaf; it is almost a bread "meme", being the most common shape of antiquity, and certainly of the classic English "cottage" or "cob" and French pain au levain loaves.

Bread destined to be crusty can also be made in a cloth-lined basket. This is the most common method of rising/proving a loaf. The cloth-lined basket will have to be made at home, but is well worth while if you intend to enter the craft, as this enables the most aesthetic loaf.

A round cane basket can easily be lined with artist's canvas. Washed first, this is simply sewn into the cane with a few stitches and will be with you forever. It is well-floured before the loaf is placed in it for proving/rising. The cloth-lined basket needs to be aired regularly to prevent the formation of mould. My ideal used to be a now-lost thick wooden bowl in which I made my first crusty breads, and such bowls are perfect for proving the crusty loaf. It is also possible to improvise with floured tea towels in plastic bowls, there are ways. Available now are "brotforms", made from thin slated wood, or plastic versions which serve as proving baskets.

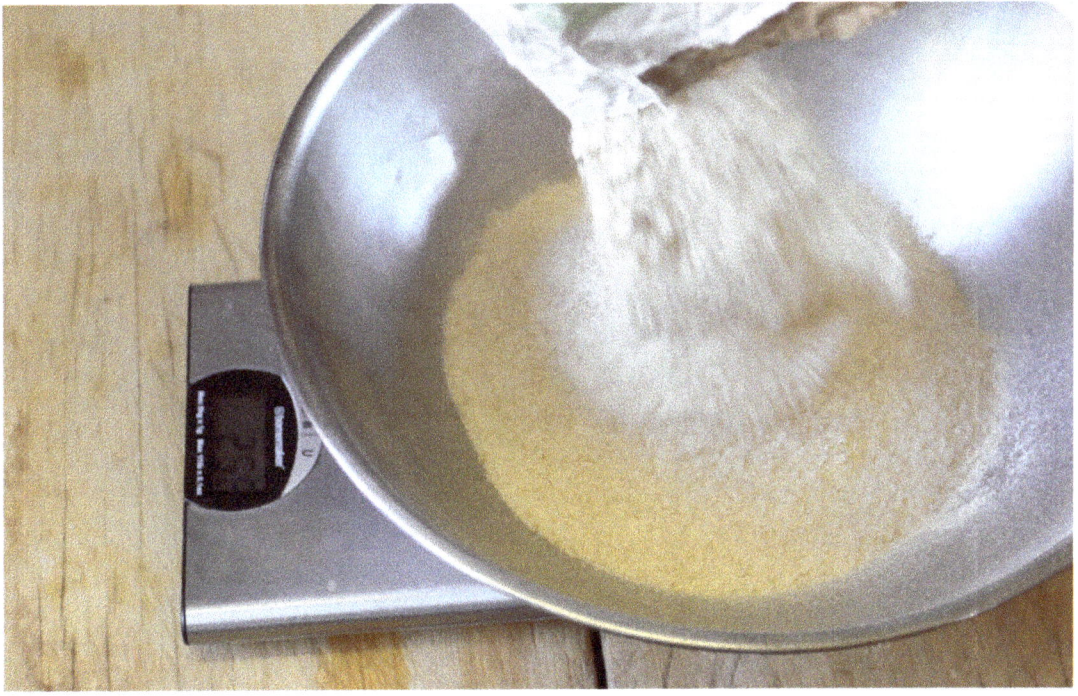

The Sourdough Loaf

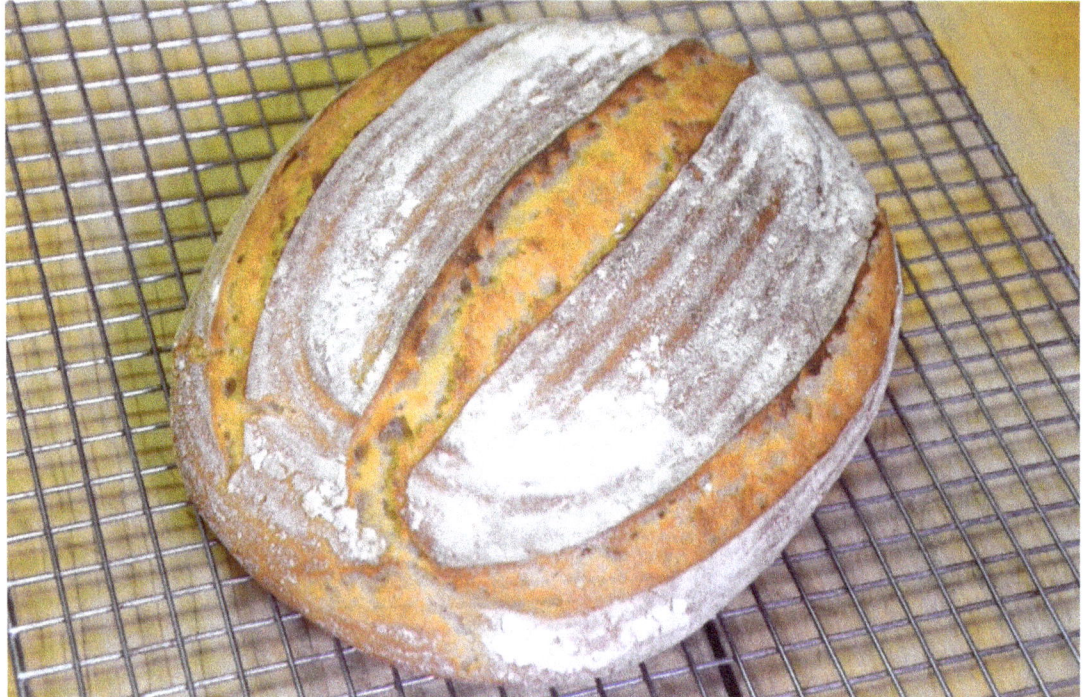

A good-solid baking tray.

For baking, the crusty loaf is turned out of its basket onto the metal tray. Make sure you obtain a tray big enough for the loaf to spread a bit, and it must fit your oven. The removable base from a metal flan tin is ideal for round loaves.

Alternatively, fanatics will purchase a bake-stone or stone tile which is heated in the oven and the loaf is turned-out on to it. This perfectly replicates the stone floor of a traditional oven and ensures the loaf gets a good " oven-spring" and is well-baked on the bottom.

Razor blades or a bread blade.

These are necessary to slash/cut the domed surface of a crusty loaf immediately prior to baking. I prefer a razor blade with tape on one side which prevents slashing the fingers along with the loaf. These cuts must be done with a seriously sharp instrument, and a knife will not do as this may tear the skin of the loaf, ruining the "look" and provoking angst.

Various professional dough-cutting blades can be purchased, including a razor-blade holder. I have tried them all and return to the hand-held razor blade, but most bakers use the thin French dough blades.

The Cloche.

This is really an extra for we fanatics. The cloche is the ultimate for home-bakers, or if you want to bake in the wilds on a camp fire. The cloche is truly ancient with many being found during excavations at Athens, and may be the original step from baking loaves such as the ancient Roman focaccia "in the ashes".

The cloche is a round stone or fired clay base which has a domed lid fitting snuggly. The base is heated in the fire, today the oven, and the crusty round loaf is turned-out on to the base. The dome is immediately placed over it and covered with hot coals, or simply shut the oven door.

The loaf billows in its own steamy enclosure. No appreciable crust is formed, as is usual in dry heat, which would reduce the oven spring. The loaf expands nicely and can be baked to completion with a fine rather than deep crust. Alternatively, in an oven, the dome is removed 15 minutes before the completion of baking, and a thin crisp crust, almost the grail of crusts forms.

A cloche may be replicated using an inverted steel or pottery bowl over the loaf as it sits on say a metal base or bakestone, and removing it before the completion of baking.

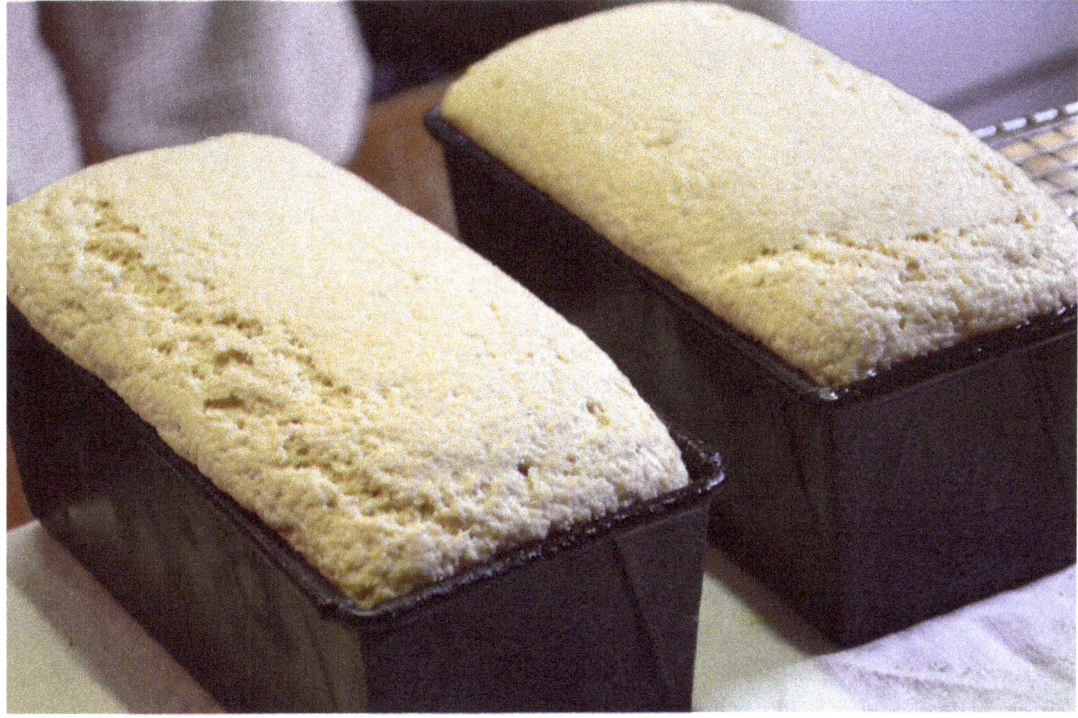

The Sourdough Loaf

Some spray water or use domestic steam cleaners to attempt the same effect, hovering expectantly at the oven door. Bowls of hot water can also be placed in the oven for a similar result, but I fear we enter the fringe of obsession, which is not a bad thing, so experiment and develop your own craft to achieve pleasing results.

Wire cooling rack.

A good wire cooling rack for the hot, just-baked loaf. This is essential as the loaf cannot be placed on a solid surface when just-baked-hot, or it will become gluggy on the bottom.

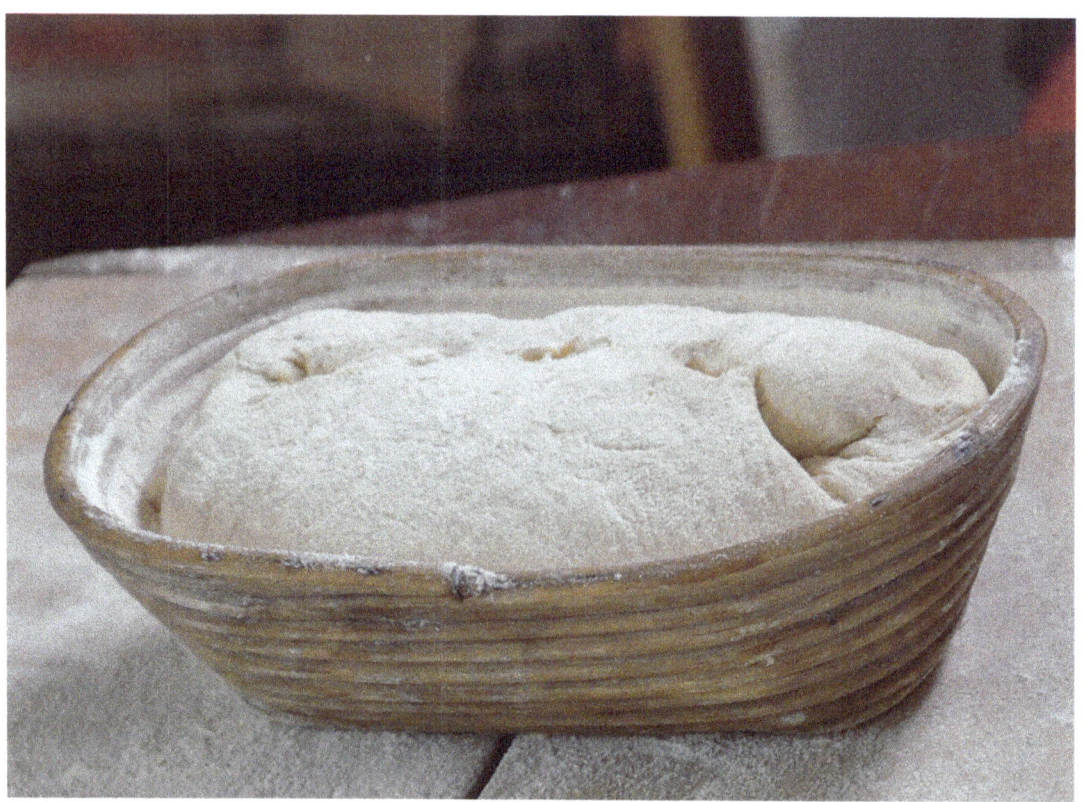

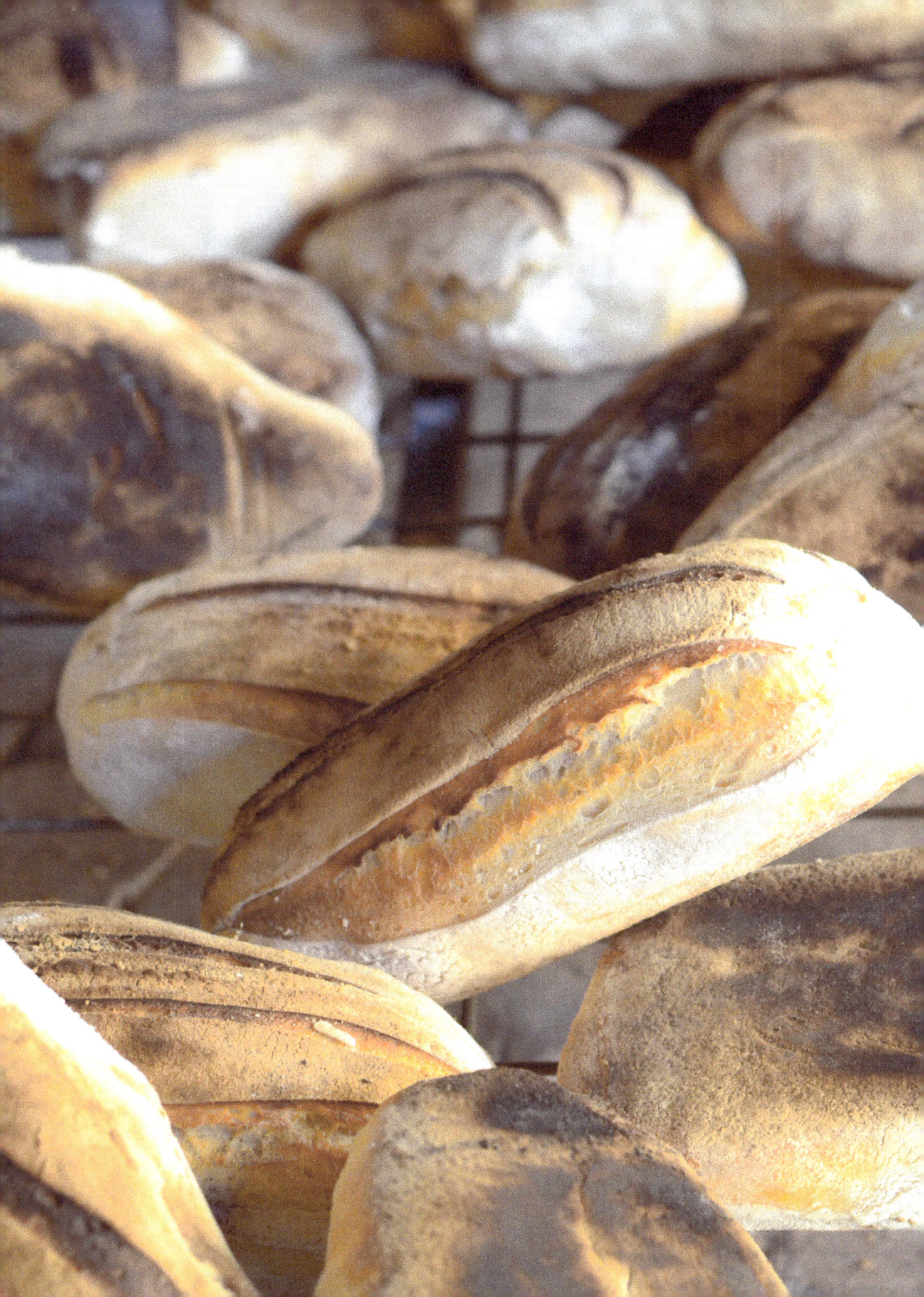

THE OVEN
Fire

Much depends upon the oven. Most simply have to deal with the oven they have, but there are very good ovens now available for home baking - or build your own.

I'm talking of the back-yard brick "igloo" or "bee-hive" oven, which dates to about 4000 BCE. Build one, cook in it and have fun; a nice alternative to a barbecue.

Home ovens, electric and gas are idiosyncratic. The temperature can vary from true, so there may be a burnt offering or a pale imitation on the first bake. These ovens are insulated to varying degrees and hold their heat, and have a more "solid" baking heat, when well-insulated.

The oven needs to be hot for crusty bread, which usually means 250°C on entry. If the oven has good solid heat and is well-insulated, the temperature may be then turned down to about 200° once the bread is in, for the rest of the baking. If the oven is a bit doubtful, maintain the high heat for about 15 minutes before turning it down, or not, but the golden rule is that the oven should be hot. A good hot oven encourages the final rise or lift, "oven-spring", and if the loaf is crusty, not tinned, high initial heat will cause the cuts/slashes on the loaf to open nicely.

The same applies to tinned breads, but the heat can be turned down soon after putting the loaves in at say 250°C, then turned down to 200°C for a lot longer than the crusty bread - usually 45 minutes to an hour if necessary. It is far better to burn the bread than under-bake it. Burnt crust can be removed (or relished) but raw-ish bread will make you ill.

Fan-forced ovens vary and can be particularly tricky, either way too hot or too cool, not true to temperature, and searing, sometimes causing the side of the loaf not exposed to the sirocco to split, while the other side is fused! Sometimes, using a pan of hot water in the bottom of the oven will moderate the blast of dry hot air...but the crust is often on the black side of brown.

Baking flatbreads on or in some post-modern barbecues is well worth trying.

These can also bake a good crusty loaf if able to be sealed with a lid, and especially if a hot bake-stone or tile is used.

The flatbread recipes are also suitable for the intrepid camper, innovating techniques on coals and "in the ashes". This is the way Australia's indigenous people made excellent breads with great skill, which became the "damper" of the European settlers. The legendary "sourdoughs" of the Alaskan and Californian gold fields always kept a funky piece of dough which they made into a bread baked in this way. It all creates an enhanced picture of camp cooking and a reality check on "damper".

Most are surely after the excellent crusty white bread, and the oven is an important part of its success. Again, the oven needs to be hot, steamy at first but crusty bread needs to be finished in dry heat, and never under-baked!

A well-made brick oven creates a lot of steam when the bread is in and the door firmly shut. This does not happen in domestic ovens, which usually leak the steam. A steamy environment is crucial to good-volume, especially for the crusty loaf. If the oven is dry/hot, a hard crust can form too quickly and the loaf cannot expand, and may burst unattractively or simply turn to stone.

Baking is hot! Always use oven-mitts or suitable gloves/cloths. When putting bowls of water in the oven to create steam, be focused as steam burns are nasty, but you will probably get a little burn as a reminder!

The oven is a womb
From which bread is born,
According to lore.
The leaven impregnates the dough
It swells
The oven is a womb
From which bread is bourne.

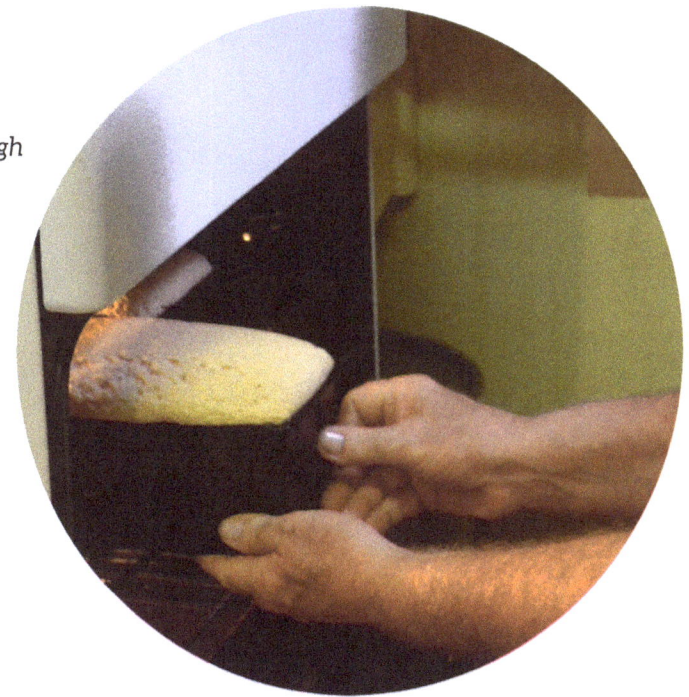

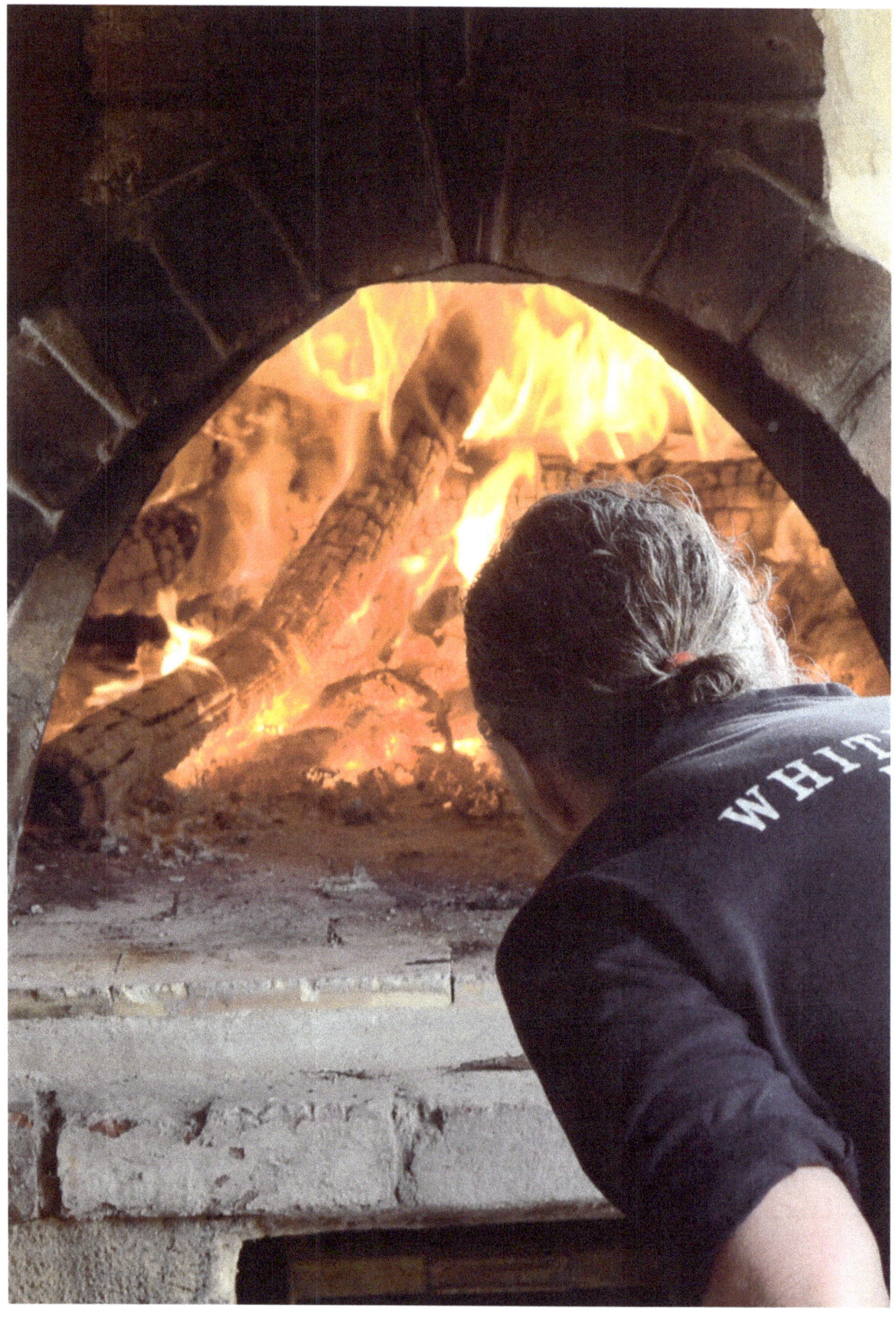

The Sourdough Loaf

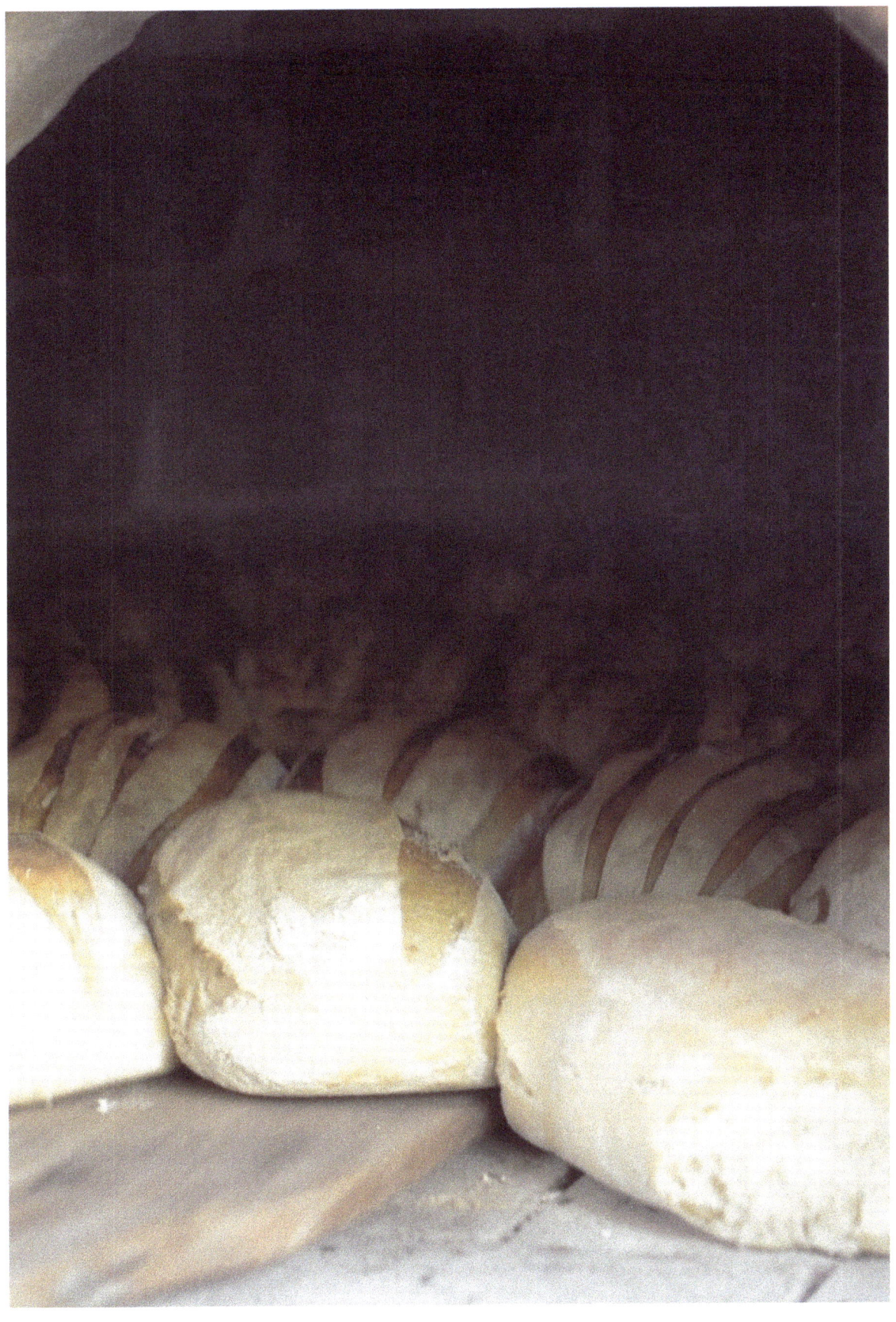

The Sourdough Loaf

TECHNIQUES AND THE 4 Ts

Time is the master, and time is the first of the "4 T's" of bread-making: time, temperature, texture and transcendence.

At the risk of sounding a little earnest, sourdough bread-making requires your attention, engagement and focus. So does making a good cake, but here we are dealing with a force of nature, not simply ingredients which if blended correctly, produce a result.

After you acquire the knack and understand the pitfalls, it is as easy as making a good cake - perhaps easier.

Time.

Firstly, presuming your leaven is ready, assemble the throng—the good-sized bowl, the slip, the wooden spoon, whisk, tea towel, plastic bag, flour, water and salt, the kit (and caboodle). Decide where you will raise (proof/prove) the bread - the not cold spot. Think it through, ensuring you have a time line. Even-though the process takes 5-6 hours for white bread, 3 ½ for wholemeal, hands on is only about 15-20 minutes. Creative scheduling will enable smooth baking.

Once you have made the initial dough, there is a one hour proof for wholemeal, or 2 hours for whiter bread. No need to hover expectantly. The next step, re-shaping and placing in the baskets or tin is just a few minutes. Then a 2-3 hour gap while the dough silently rises in its warm nest. Finally, putting the bread in the oven. All of this easily fits into a domestic schedule, even a creative or professional one.

No time to make bread? Are you sure? Granted you need to be in the vicinity and in the "zone", but it's not much in the scheme of things. An inevitable domestic day could at least have a loaf/loaves of bread as its reward whilst multi-tasking.

Bakers easily handle dough, are deft and dextrous - enviably to the home baker. It is experience, but a core of that is the speed at which the baker's hand touches and leaves the dough. The hand rarely lingers, leaving no time for the dough to stick. There really is minimal handling in these methods anyway, but advanced home bakers will want to knead, round and shape with a deft quick hand as a key to success. Do not linger when handling dough as sticky edgy sourdoughs stick. Another key to the time involved in handling doughs is to flour your hands. Perhaps have a bowl of flour "handy" to dip into.

The time frame for making a basic white crusty loaf is 6 ½ hours from when you begin the dough. It is quite strict as the loaf will over-rise or over-proof quite rapidly as it achieves maximum ripeness and will become softer, flowing, unable to oven-spring, or to burst aesthetically through skilful slashes and achieve golden-brown glory. No, it will flow and be flat and a bit sour, the cuts staying blind. Under-baked it would be what I call "sour, damp and heavy".

Maximum ripeness and readiness for the oven is the most important time to closely observe. Bakers call this either "over-proof", gone too far, or "under-proof", not ready for the oven. Proof is the perfect time and stage at which the loaf usually must be baked. Bakers may take the loaf "under-proof" and then slash deeply so it will burst within the cuts and expand attractively, but they will ensure that the loaf is "ripe"—well fermented. This is manipulation of time done skilfully.

Traditional bakers always used the terms "ripe" and "green" when referring to fermenting dough. Think of the best fruit you have ever eaten with all the perfect qualities of sweetness, tart balance, flavour and aroma characteristic of that fruit, it would be my Father's apricots nectarines or tomatoes for me. This is the quality of "ripe" when referring to a dough.

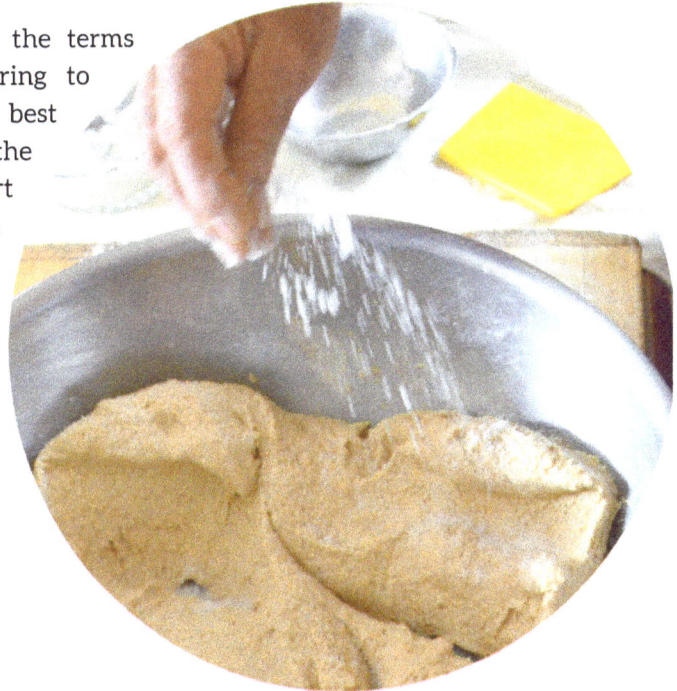

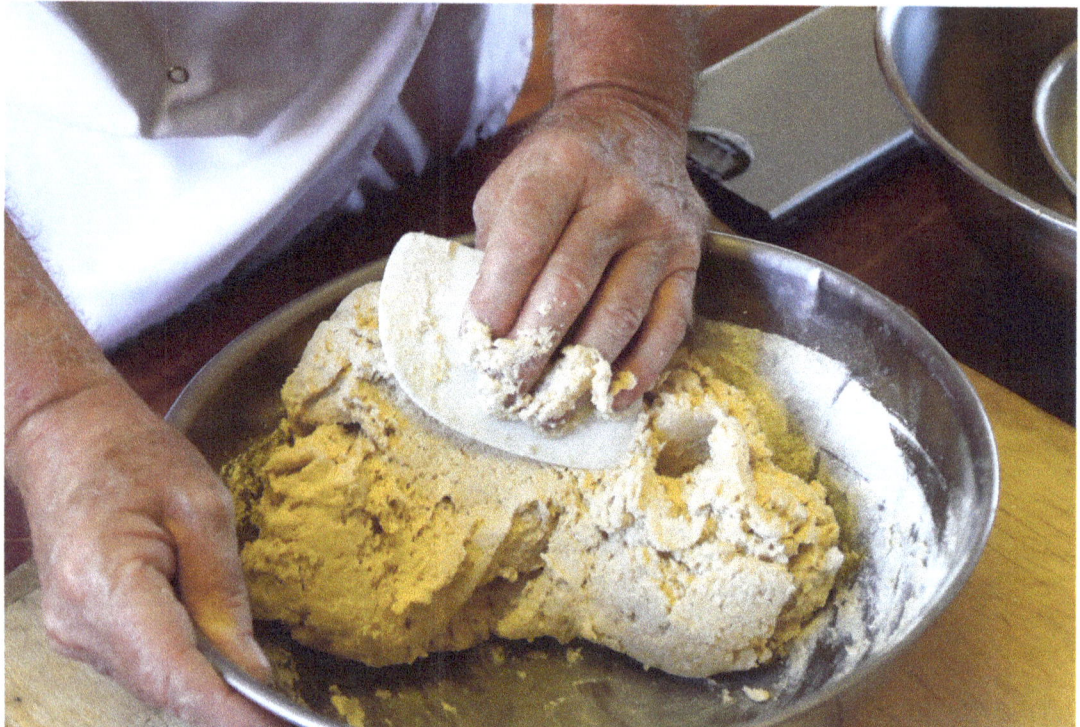

For a sourdough, this means the sweetness of yeasts dominating the action, just before the bacteria usher in decay in the fruit and the dough. "Green" clearly means the dough is not ready, not sweet enough, and needs to ripen further.

Temperature.

Time and temperature inter-react significantly. Usually a "regular" time frame is known, for the loaf to rise, but a drop in temperature in the process will cause the rising to slow down. Similarly, a loaf can be warmed in what bakers call a "proover", or a warm nest, to accelerate the rise, reducing the rising time. A warm place is required in cold climates and winter as the loaf will be slow to rise unless it is kept warm.

Bakers also manipulate time and temperature by intentionally cooling even chilling a loaf so it rises very slowly. Leaving bread to rise over-night in a refrigerated space achieves this aim. When the bread is warmed in the morning, it rises again and can be baked, sometimes with spectacular results as the many tiny pockets of air which develop as the loaf slumbers, suddenly expand and create a holey texture if the dough is soft, making a very fashionable-looking loaf.

A thermometer is the standard tool for monitoring dough and water temperature. I rarely if ever use one, which is fine for me, but most bakers do, and it will help you to gain the "feel" anyway. Doughs below 23°C are on the cold side and will be slow to activate. Ideal dough temperature for these methods is 25-27°C, and 30°C is alright under a different algorithm of the 4Ts. There is always an interplay of the divine Ts which any baker can manipulate craftily.

Bakers with a more "mechanised state of sensation" also measure flour temperature as well as water temperature. The average of these temperatures should be the temperature you want, tempered by the ambient temperature. Using ice-cold water in a dough, which is done in the tropics and on an Australian or Spanish 40°C baking day, is also a delaying procedure.

On such a hot day, the dough will increase in temperature so fast from the ambient heat, it will rapidly ferment back to a liquid if warm water is used, for example, causing the dough to simply disintegrate as it is handled.

As an indicator of the importance of ambient temperature, in the north of India, the "unleavened" wheat dough for chapatti is actually leavening within minutes of being made, because the ambient temperature and humidity is so high and the flour and water are also warm, all initiating spontaneous fermentation.

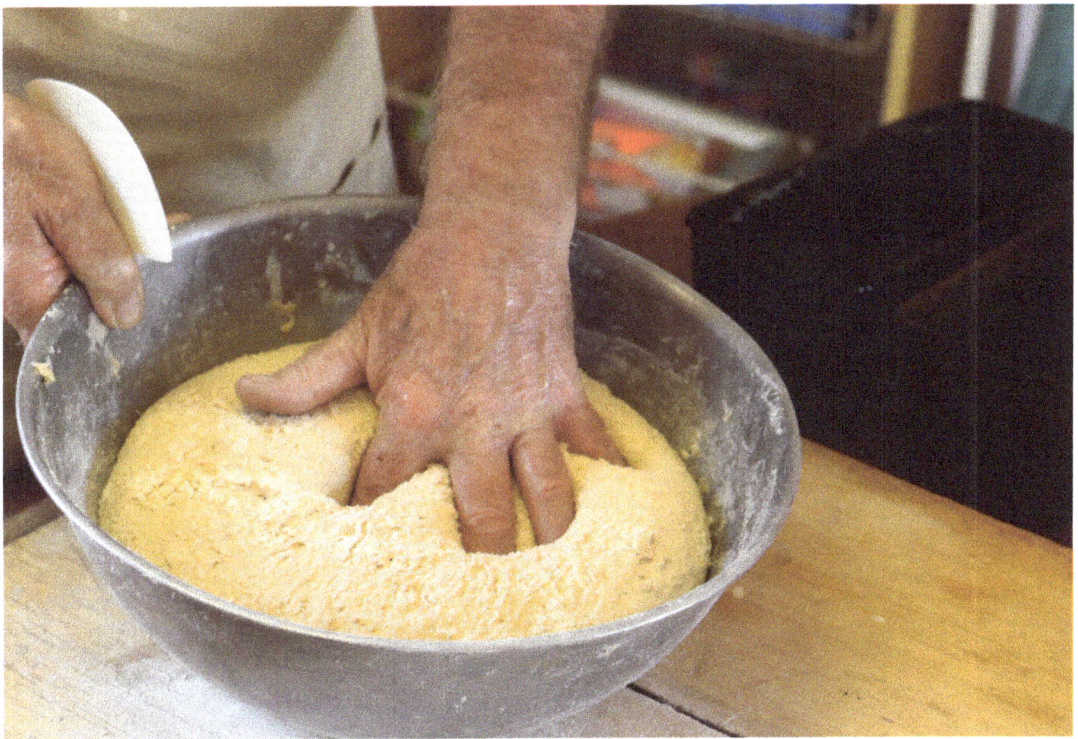

The Sourdough Loaf

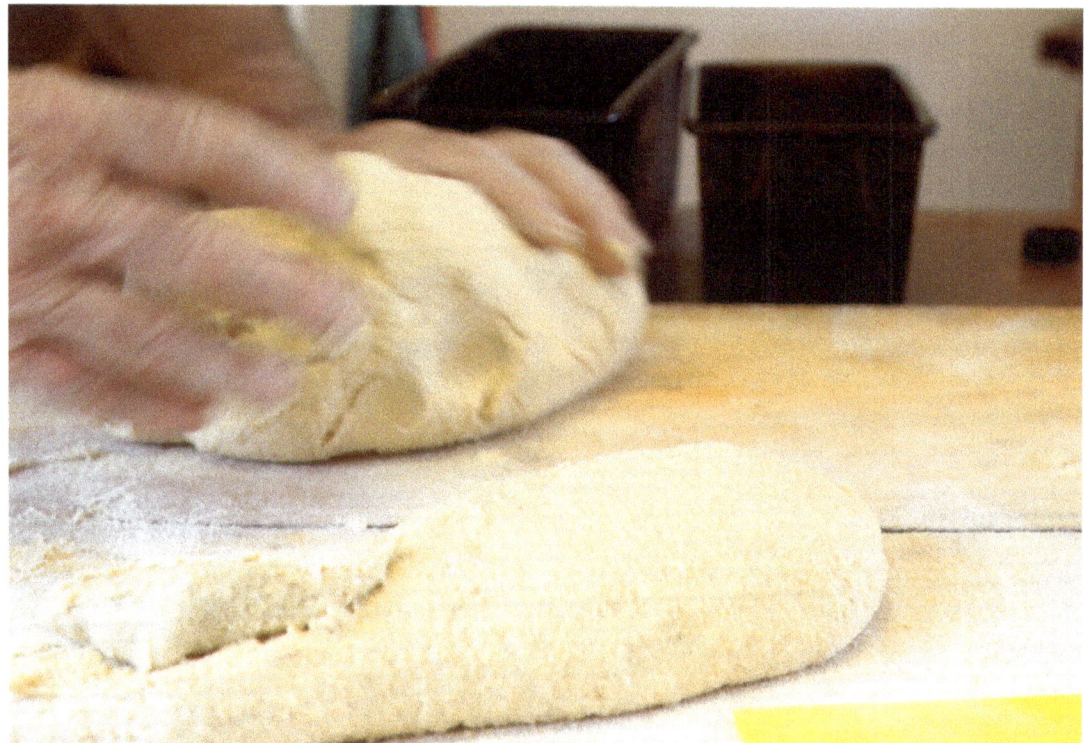

If the dough is about 10kg, which is average for a chapatti maker (walla), the dough being cut off gradually for each piece ferments before your eyes, and by the end, the chapatti are quite lacy and flaky, also very delicious being ghee-tinged and tasty from the stone-ground khorassan wheat commonly used, especially in the villages.

Similarly a dough in an English winter just doesn't move, if made and proved at ambient temperature. "Bread requires warmth".

The effect of temperature is also why the style of bread and the baker's craft in a hot climate differs from the Euro-Anglosphere norm. In hot countries the norm is flat breads, as dough for basketed or tinned breads becomes un-handleable so rapidly that the dough breaks down before it can rise sufficiently to fill the basket or tin, and by this stage is quite sour. The flat breads in these countries, where wheat originates, are the original bread.

As you can see from this inter-play, a sourdough becomes softer even flowing as it ferments or proves and ripens. This is because of the extensive bio-activity of the dough as the microbiome actually digests the dough and importantly as the gluten superstructure is broken down. In a fully fermented, ripe dough, all the gluten has been rendered into smaller particles, and basically there is no gluten left.

Most sourdoughs will not reach this sort of texture, as bakers (especially, amateur bakers) need some structure. Flatbreads can easily achieve this state and are a good choice for those who would like the bread to contain minimal or no gluten.

Skilled bakers with a wood-fired oven can manipulate this softening of the dough to good effect. The quality of the heat in a well-insulated stone or brick oven is such that, when hot (300°C), a fully fermented conventionally shaped loaf can be baked. These disconcertingly collapse when placed in the oven from the peel (or "bat"), yet after only 20 minutes baking, are reborn phoenix-like, glowing with burnished tones, massively inflated with a holey texture and substantial shaley crisp crust. This is the very best of sourdough wheat bread. It is a fine correspondence of the 4 Ts, however all must be "in time" or the loaf chars or does not recover its volume.

Texture.

The inter-reaction of time, temperature, and texture is important. If a refrigerated dough has a very soft texture, perhaps made with more water than usual, the baker can achieve massively cavernous, alveolated interior structure, "wondrous faery architecture", by cooling it and extending time (over-night). This texture is much desired and can only be achieved by this or similar methods - but is ruined if transcendence, unexpected power failure, or a failure to refrigerate it occurs.

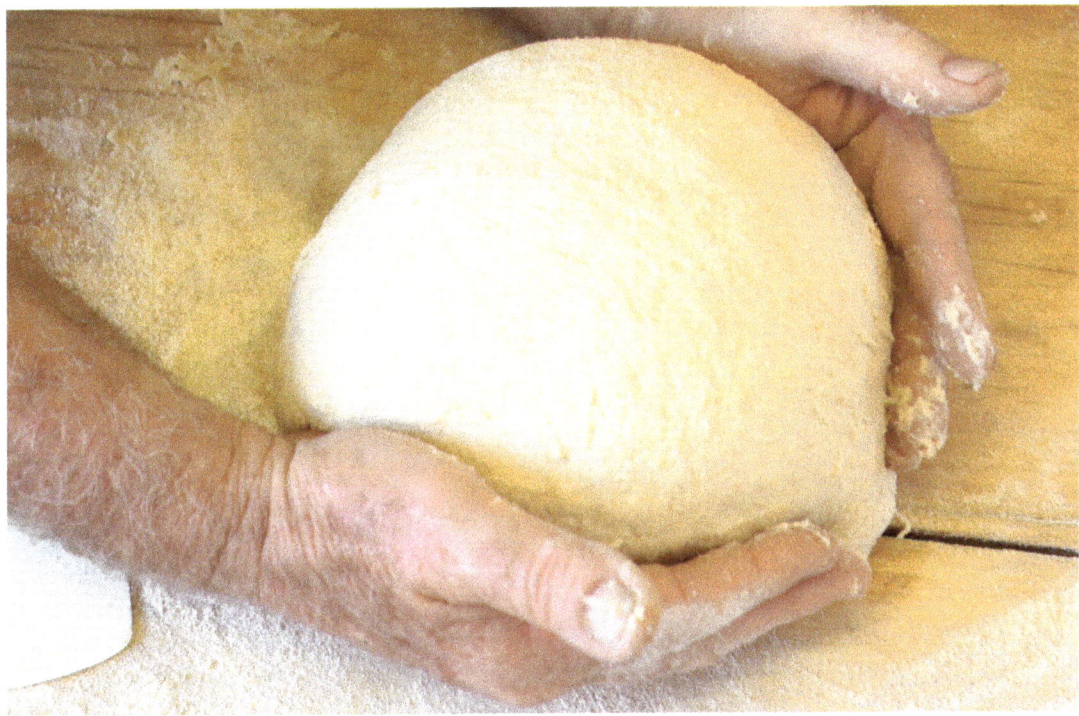

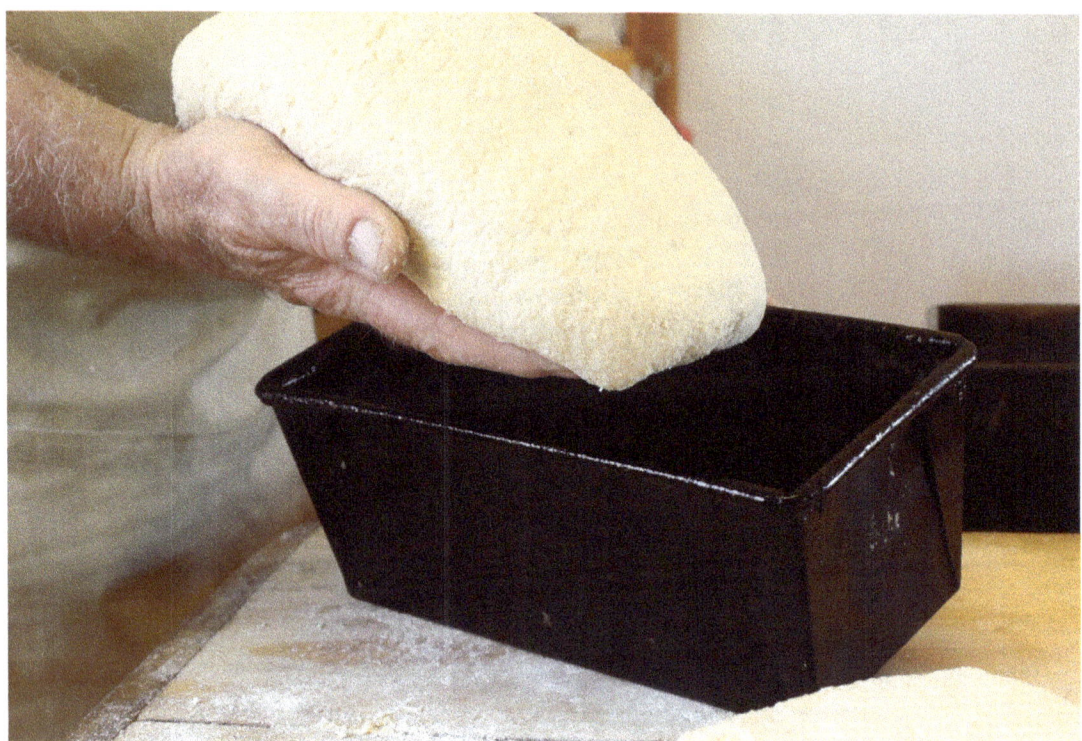

If the dough had been made with a firmer texture, the faery architecture of caverns and caves can not be achieved. The loaf would be "blind" - close-textured.

The texture of a dough should always be softer than harder. If the dough will not yield to your touch, more water needs to be added to soften or loosen it so it can easily activate and rise. The final baked texture will also be better. If a dough is made "tight" or "hard" the final texture will be close. Further, it will not achieve oven-spring and may burst un-attractively and form a hard crust, edible surely, but un-remarkable.

The texture of rye bread is at odds to wheat bread texture. 100% rye dough will be sticky, difficult to handle and a mess. This is where hands and bench must be lightly floured to enable handling. A full rye sour, once mixed and "clear", with no unmixed flour, should be quickly shaped, rolled in flour for ease of handling and tinned without further ado. The dough will sort itself out in the tin, relax and rise slowly looking more like dough than a mess.

Mixing technique.

Some of you will have a dough-mixing device, which makes mixing easy and less strenuous. The first step when making a dough is to put the water in and then add the leaven. Mix on low speed for a few minutes, with the whisk attachment until the mix is frothy and (usually) smells of beer, which is a good sign that the yeasts are active. If mixing in a bowl, follow the same procedure, using a whisk before adding the flour and salt.

The dough may be mixed and kneaded in the same, suitable bowl. I rarely place the dough on the bench for kneading unless it is a crusty white, which does require a workout.

By withholding some of the flour, that is making a wet-sticky dough with just ¾ of the flour added, the dough may be simply stirred with the wooden spoon, allowing gluten strands to form readily and for rapid hydration. Leave this to stand for 5 minutes and surprisingly, it has virtually kneaded itself with long, muscley strands of gluten evident. Allowing the dough to relax is a very important strategy in bread making. Dough needs a rest.

Add the remaining flour, mix it and knead slowly, spinning the bowl as you work. Almost magically a nice stable springy dough will form. This is enough kneading usually for a homely bread. Granted, more kneading may be needed for strong flour doughs, but again, resting the dough between bouts of kneading is important. If you feel the need, go ahead, knead and develop a more sophisticated structure of artisanal standard.

Mixing and kneading is really easy and not extremely strenuous, especially if one remains or becomes calm, no need for performance anxiety. I like to get out of the way and let the bread make itself, which may sound trite until this rhythm reveals itself as you make bread more often.

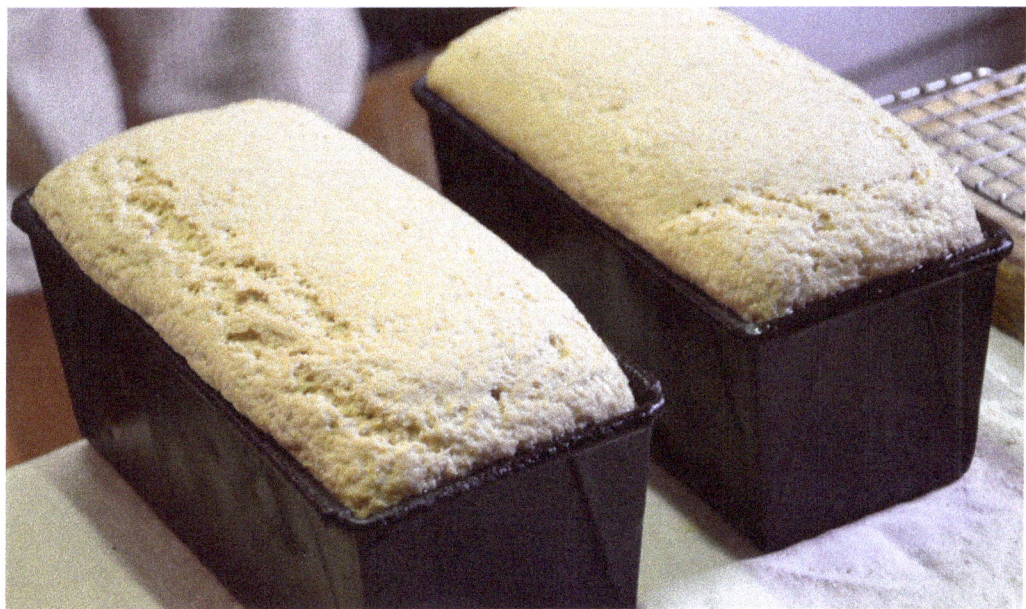

The Sourdough Loaf

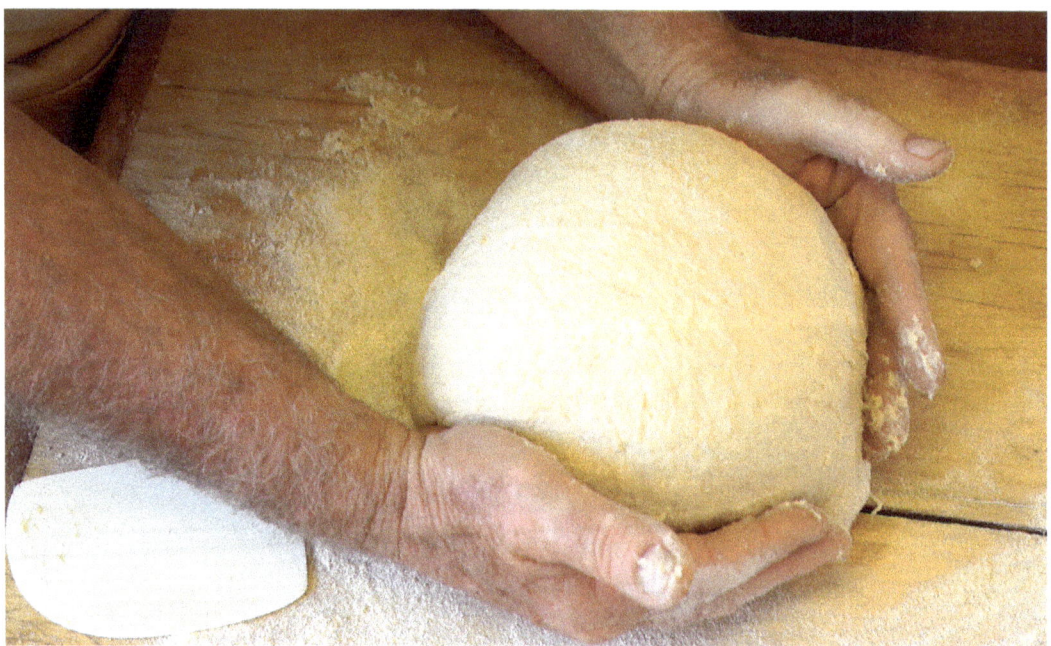

Shaping.

Before the loaf can be placed in a tin or a basket or folded cloth (couche), it has to be transformed from an amorphous mass into some sort of shape. This is known as "shaping" or "moulding".

For commercial bakers this is a necessity to provide some uniformity. The Zeppelin loaves must be shaped that way if they are to rise in the cloths, and similarly, a nice tin bread will rise very un-aesthetically if just dumped in the tin and allowed to burst up through unsealed joints and cracks. Shaping is one of the "art" bits in "artisan".

The most basic shape which should be mastered by home bakers is the ball shape. From this shape, all others can be formed with a little folding. The aim of shaping, is to produce a "uniform density", which will not happen if the dough piece is simply dumped into its resting place.

If dumped and not shaped, there may be heavy, dense areas, with some more aerated than others, which may not affect those of you simply thrilled to have made an edible loaf, but as time goes on, you will want it to look a little "artisanal", aesthetic even, a bit like the one of the groovy breads in the sourdough bakery.

A sourdough storyboard

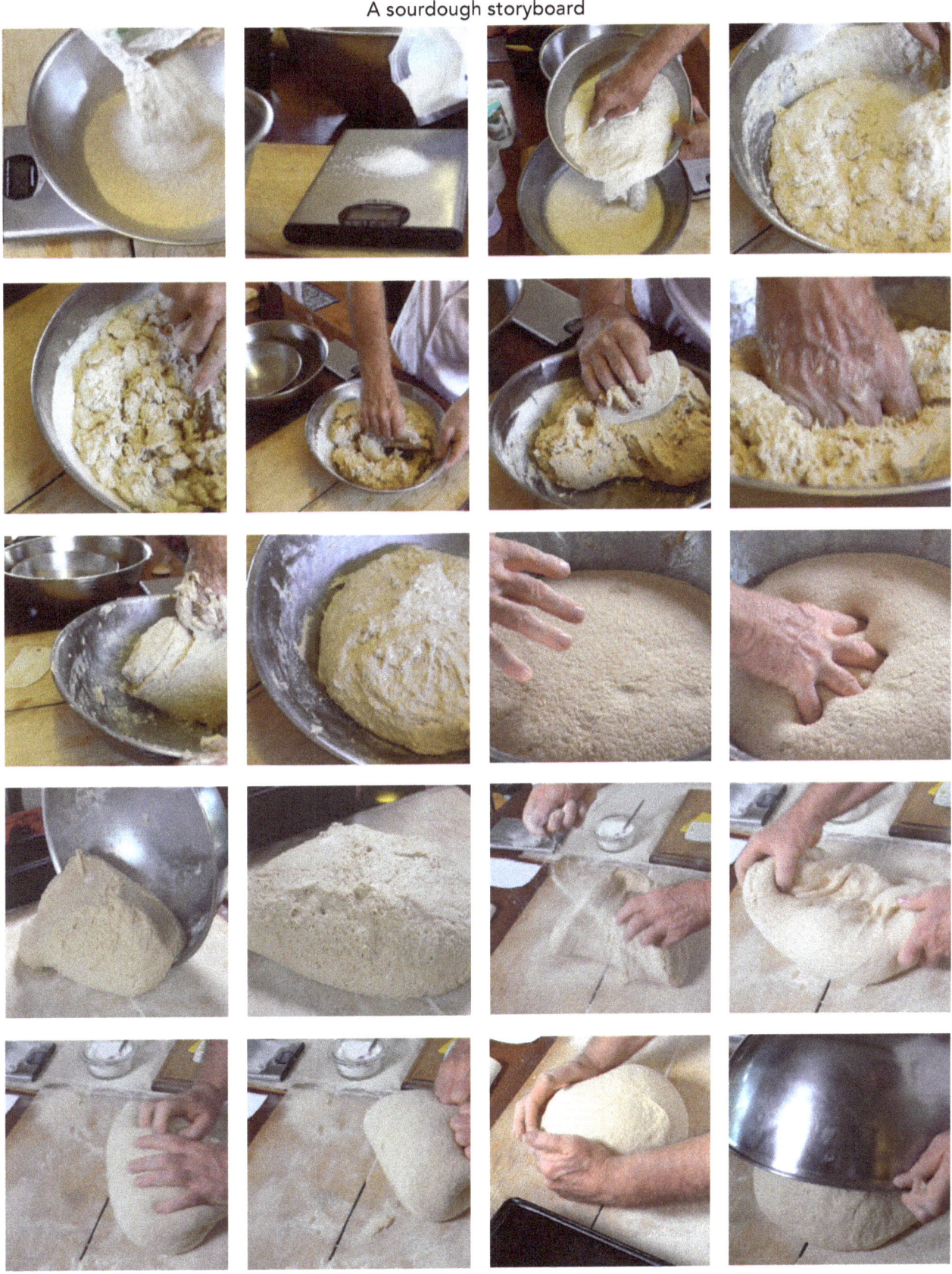

Shaping requires a degree of compression, to ensure the dough doesn't just flow into an irregular mass. A little scary, but simply try to form the dough mass into a ball, a smooth ball, however you can.

Tucking the edges of your palm under the bottom of the piece, try to form an exterior skin by stretching, drawing the dough around itself, pulling it closer towards you as it moves across the kneading surface, coaxing it into a smooth ball shape, and "rounding" it. Move your hands quickly, deftly, don't dwell on the piece of dough or it will stick.

If it isn't working, stop and allow the piece to relax before trying again. This is important as the piece of dough must be plastic, not tensed through repeated attempts to make it conform. The best way to achieve this rounding is to watch a skilled baker, or get someone to show you. Once acquired, you won't lose the skill.

By whatever means, once you have this round ball of dough, it can be dredged with flour and placed in a basket. To make it into a long loaf, let the ball relax, flatten it slightly and fold it over itself to form a log. Avoid using too much flour as you shape or the seams will not meld. Similarly shape a loaf destined for the tin, with seams underneath and a nice smooth top ready to dome.

Moulding/shaping very tacky or sticky doughs destined for extreme alveolation, like many fashionable loaves today, is difficult and requires practice and importantly, speed. The hand must not dwell at all but perform the shaping with extreme dexterity. In this case, the baker's slip (scraper), is vital as it can flip the dough into shape with little compression and it will not stick to your hands.

A loaf destined for the tin needs to be well rounded a few times to expel gas and provide the required uniform texture.

A sourdough storyboard (cont...)

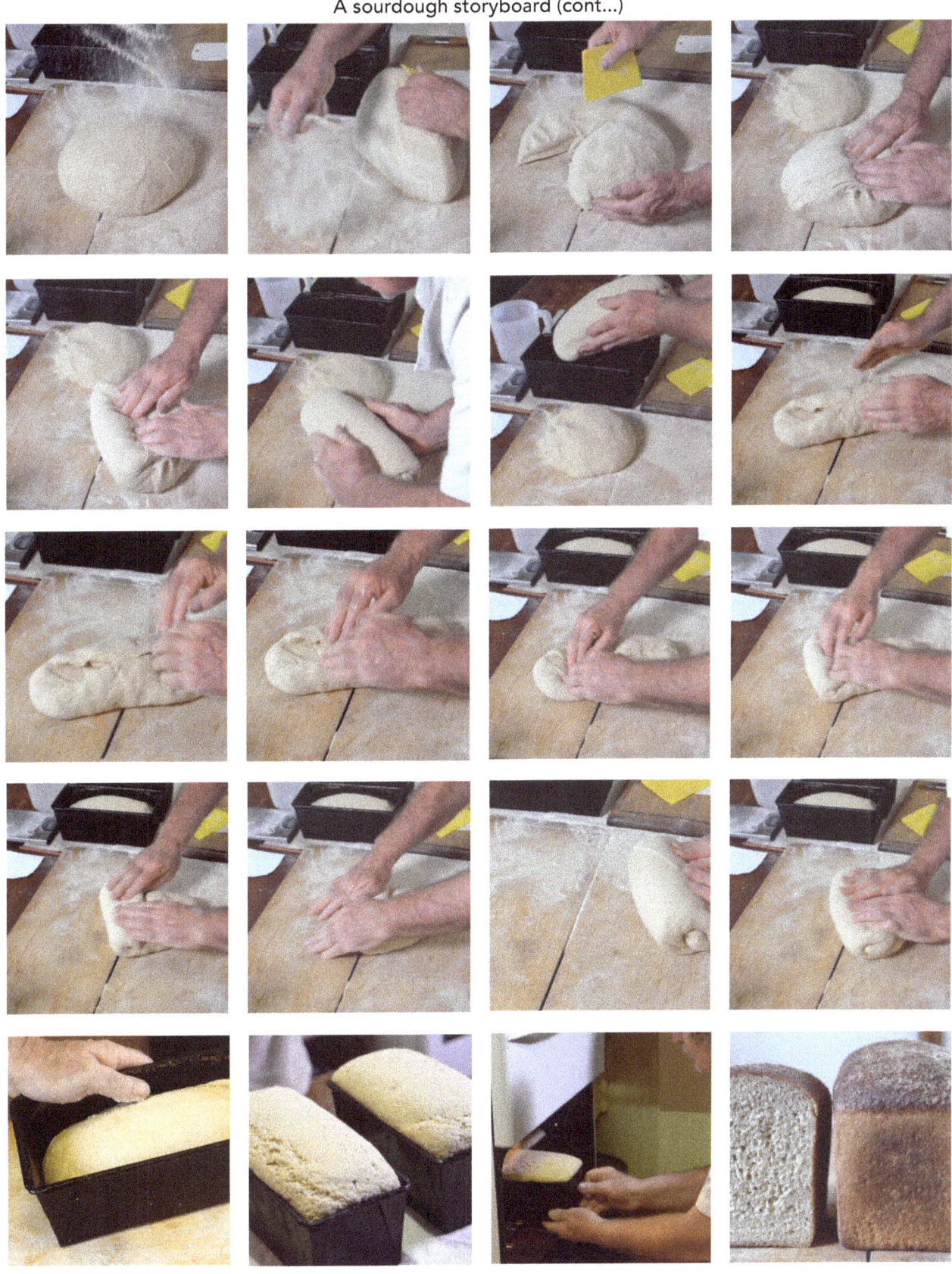

The Sourdough Loaf

METHOD FOR A CRUSTY BREAD.

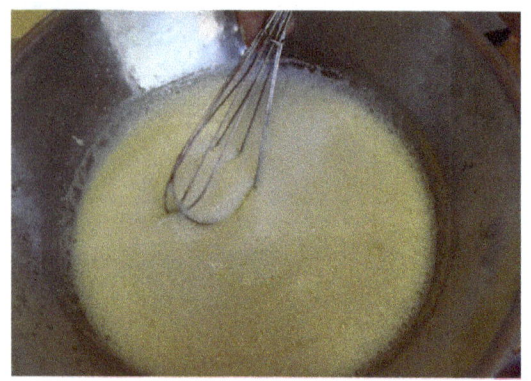

This crusty bread template describes the method for making a white crusty bread, but it can be applied to any of the crusty bread recipes.

1.   Dissolve the salt in a little of the water and set aside. Mix the rest of the water with the leaven and whisk it until a bit frothy.

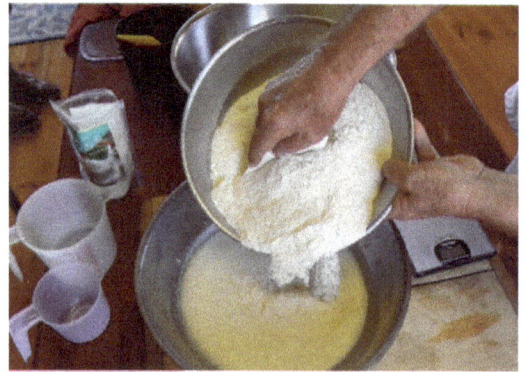

2.   Add the flour, and using either a dough mixer or wooden spoon, mix until it starts to come together, then add the salt water.

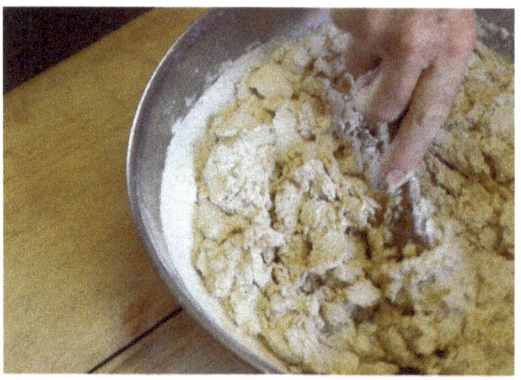

3.   Continue to mix with the spoon until the dough comes together, rotating the bowl as you work or turn out onto a lightly floured surface, merely dusted, and commence working and kneading. This isn't really easy as the dough is a little sticky, so flour your hands and use a bakers slip to keep turning, folding and working the dough.

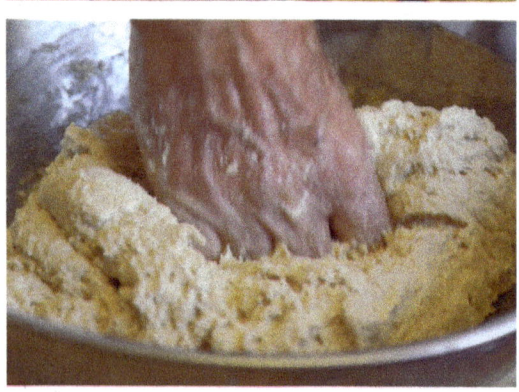

4.   The kneading takes about 5 minutes to form a less sticky, coherent dough. If the kneading is too difficult because of stickiness, dust some flour on the surface to make it easier… or use a spatula in the mixer to encourage the dough to form, dusting lightly with flour.

The Sourdough Loaf

METHOD FOR A CRUSTY BREAD CONT.

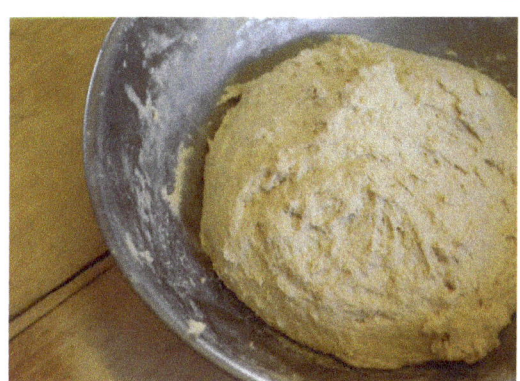

5. Form the dough into a round and roll/round it to establish a sphere . Place it in a lightly floured bowl, cover with a cloth and plastic to seal. Leave it in a not-cold spot, 25°C is ideal, for 2 hours.

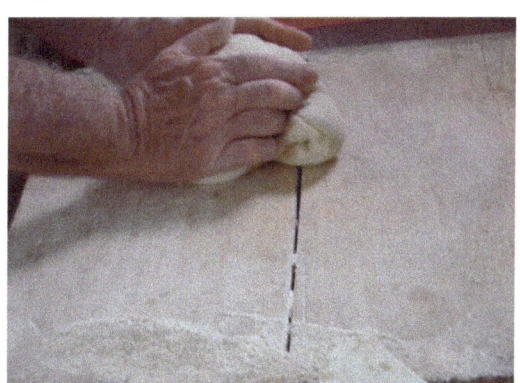

6. Dust a little flour on a working surface and turn the loaf out and with floured hands again, fold it a few times and work into a nice round.

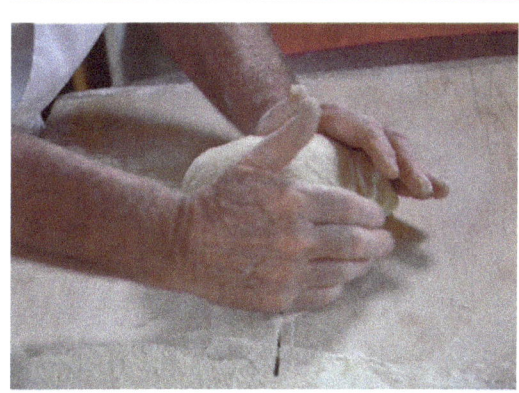

7. It should come together and "muscle-up" with a skin like a balloon.

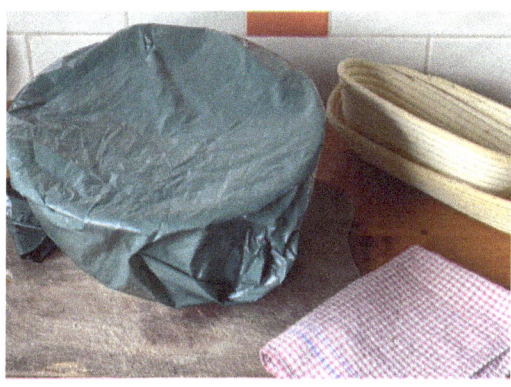

8. Cover with the cloth and plastic and leave for another hour, especially if the flour is strong.

METHOD FOR A CRUSTY BREAD CONT.

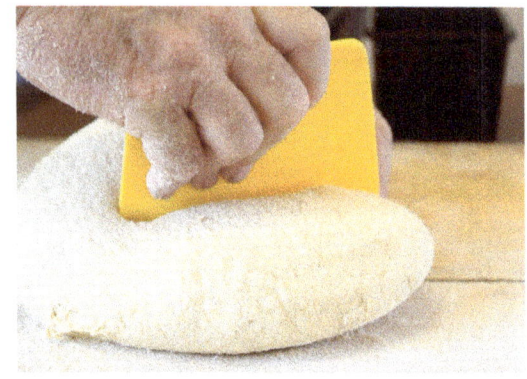

9.   Empty the dough onto a lightly floured board and divide using the baker's slip. Round each again, rolling them into torpedo shapes or rounds (ball shape), depending on the basket.

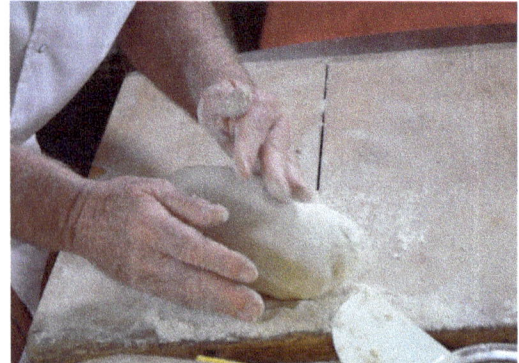

10.   Roll the shape in flour and place in the well-floured basket/banneton/brotform, with the smooth round surface down in the basket and the seam/navel uppermost.

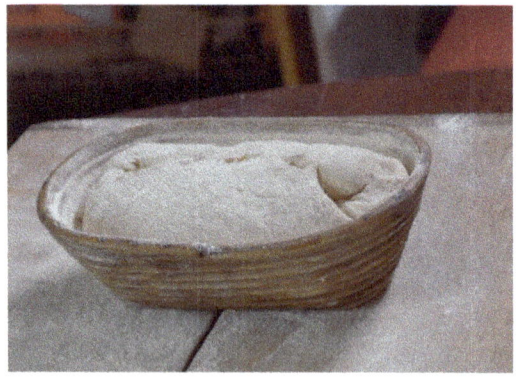

11.   Cover with the cloth and plastic bag. The cloth will absorb moisture ensuring the loaf doesn't stick to the basket.

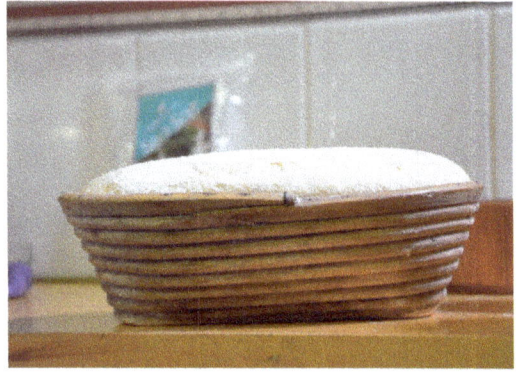

12.   This will then rise/prove for 2½ hours more, by which time it should be well-risen and billowing.

METHOD FOR A CRUSTY BREAD CONT.

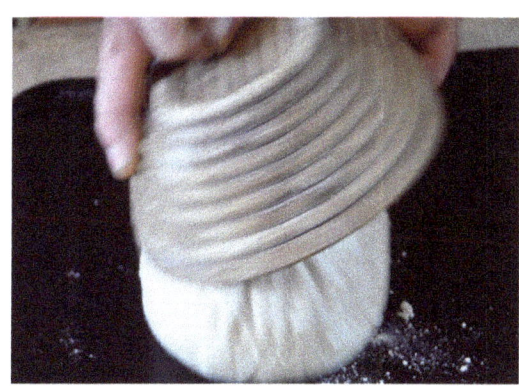

13. Pre-heat the oven to 250° C. The baking sheet or stone should be pre-heated in the oven. Have on hand a very sharp blade.

14. Turn the loaf out on to the baking sheet/stone and deftly slash it, not too deep, more slicing the skin. A cross or "hashtag" is a usual slash for a round loaf and diagonal slashes, perhaps one long cut for an oblong or torpedo (zeppelin) shape. If slashing it seems too hard, don't slash the loaf, just let it burst where it will.

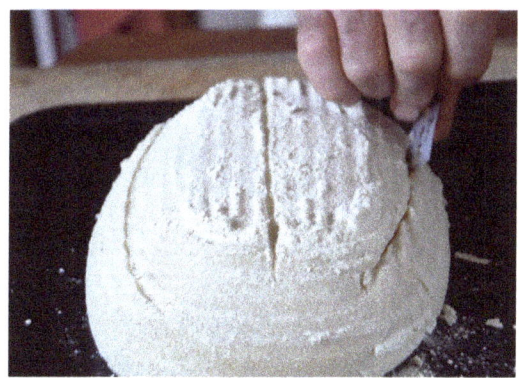

15. Reduce the heat to 200°C as soon as the loaf is in. The dough size described in the following recipes will take 20-25 minutes to bake, depending on the oven. If you like it crusty, turn the oven off leaving the loaf in for 10 more minutes with the door open.

16. Alternatively and for max crust, bake at 200°C for 30 minutes. It should rise nicely in the oven, opening the cuts/slashes attractively and have some good colour. If using a metal tray, remove it after 10 minutes of baking time.

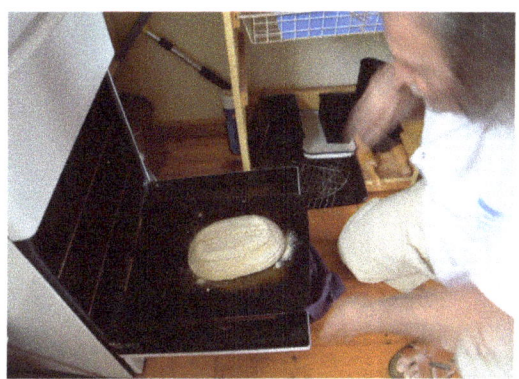

17. Invert the baked loaf and tap it for the hollow sound, and if you aren't convinced, return to the oven for 5 minutes more. When baked, put it on a cooling rack to cure and cool.

Unlike a wholemeal, this loaf only requires a few hours to cool and can be greedily sliced or torn and eaten while still warm, deliciously with good butter.

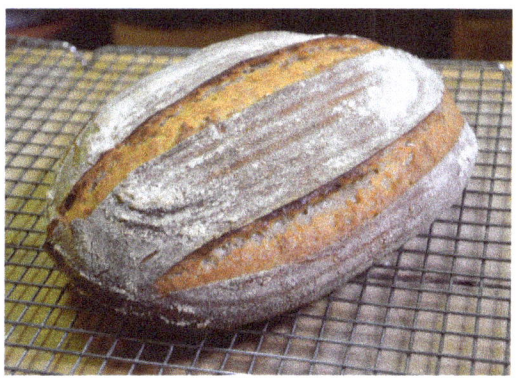

METHOD FOR A TIN BREAD.

This tin bread template describes the method for making a wholemeal tin bread, but it can be applied to any of the tin bread recipes.

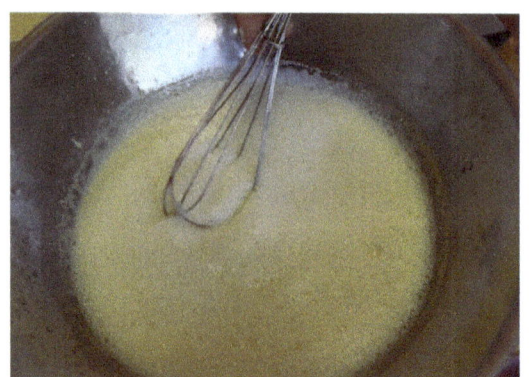

1. Dissolve the salt in some of the water. In a large bowl, mix the leaven and most of the water, and whisk until frothy.

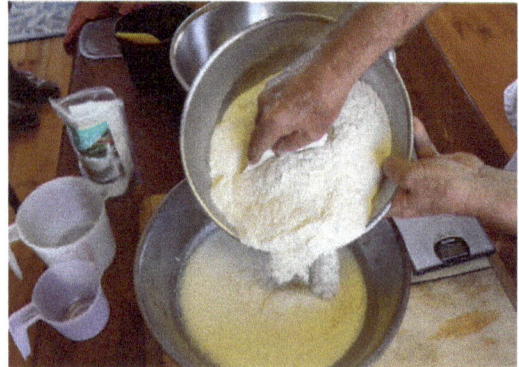

2. Add the flour, and unless using a dough mixer, mix with a wooden spoon until it starts to come together, then add the salt water.

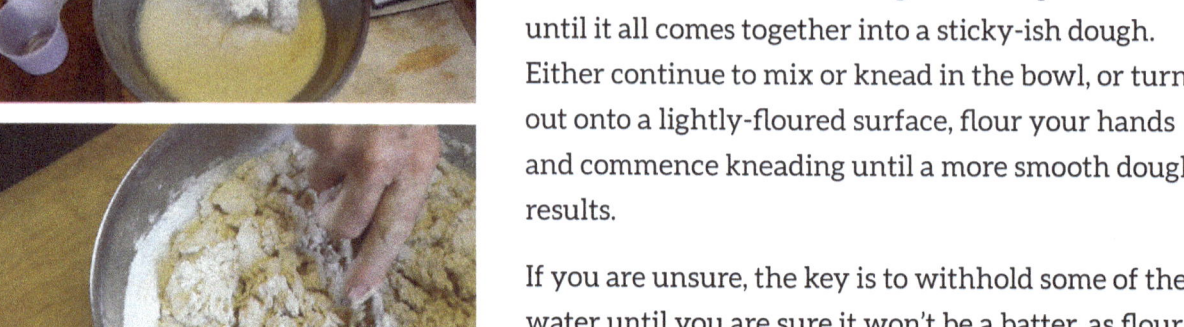

3. Mix well with a strong wooden spoon or mixer until it all comes together into a sticky-ish dough. Either continue to mix or knead in the bowl, or turn it out onto a lightly-floured surface, flour your hands and commence kneading until a more smooth dough results.

If you are unsure, the key is to withhold some of the water until you are sure it won't be a batter, as flours differ in their water absorption. Water can be added half way through the kneading, this is a very forgiving process. Ensure you are satisfied with the dough … it must not be so sticky it sticks unrepentantly to the surface, so add more flour if you think necessary, but err on the side of stickiness or softness if unsure.

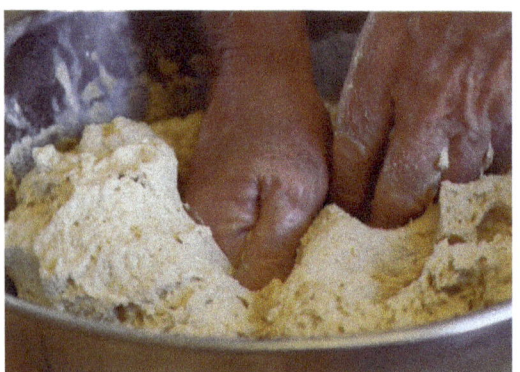

A wholemeal will usually absorb some of the stickiness and be surprisingly handleable when it comes to be shaped.

The Sourdough Loaf

METHOD FOR A TIN BREAD CONT.

There is no rush or competition for kneading excellence, just keep the dough moving, even simply rolling it to absorb all the water and slowly, rhythmically, form it into a ball and work it.

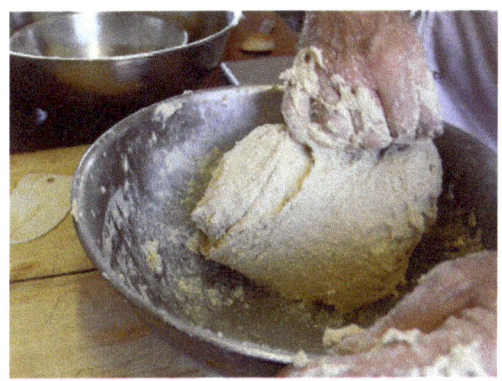

4. When you are satisfied that it has become smoother and a little less sticky, and is "clear" which means no shaggy lumps or bits of un-incorporated flour in it, place it in a bowl, cover with a cotton cloth (tea towel). Put the lot in a plastic bag, and set in a warm spot (at least not cold) for 1 hour to rise if using a soft flour, or up to 2 hours if you have a very strong wholemeal flour. This is called "bulk proof".

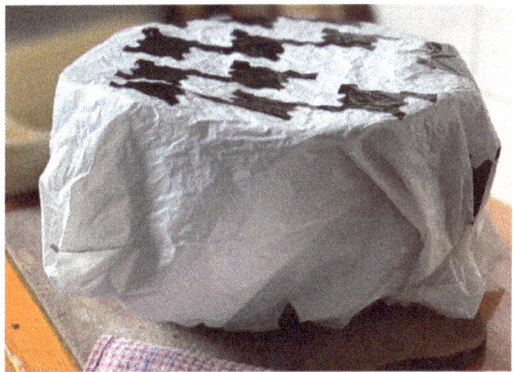

5. After one hour it should be slightly inflated, bulging, if not, wait 15 minutes, but certainly no more than one hour if using a soft wholemeal, or 2 hours for a strong wholemeal.

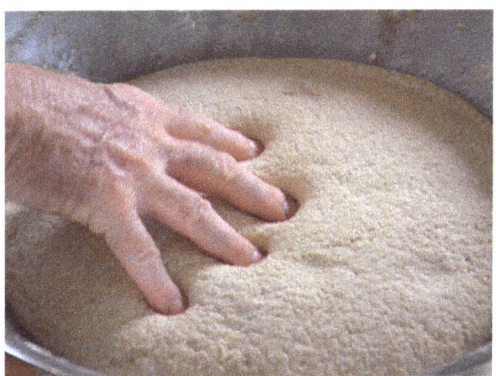

6. Turn it out onto a lightly floured surface and work it gently by briefly re-kneading, and shape or roll into a ball. A strong wholemeal, muscley, will benefit from a thorough re-kneading followed by a rest. Depending on the quantities made, the dough can be baked as two tin breads, a tin and a crusty or a loaf and some flatbreads or pizza bases, it's up to you.

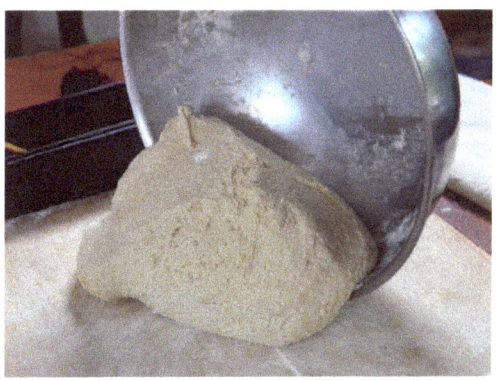

METHOD FOR A TIN BREAD CONT.

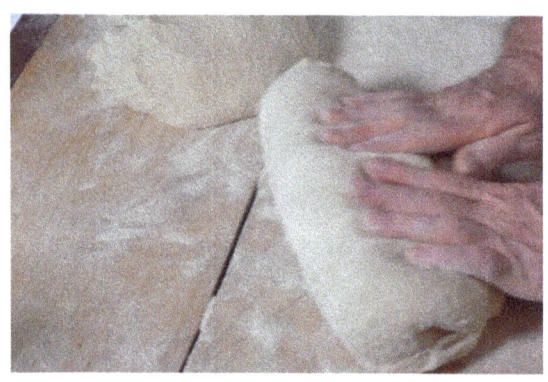

7. Divide the ball and if making two tinned breads, roll each into an oblong or tube, so there is a seam on the bottom.

8. Place in a pre-warmed well-oiled tin with the seam on the bottom, smooth surface on top.

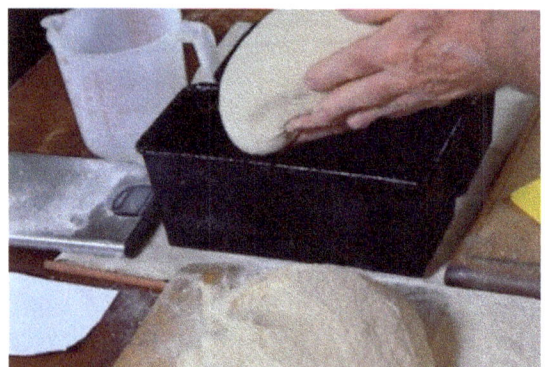

9. Cover as before and keep in a warm spot to rise. A strong wholemeal will take 2 to 2 ½ hours to rise completely. This is shown by small holes breaking the surface or a fissure or two. A soft wholemeal will reach its zenith after two hours, any further fermenting with a soft flour and the loaf may collapse or have a crack through the middle when baked.

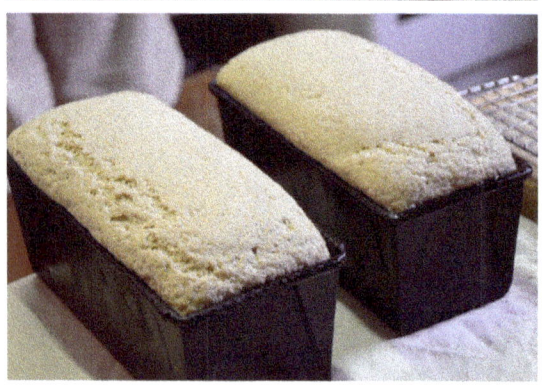

10. Depending on the size chosen, bake bigger loaves at 200°C for 45-50 minutes, smaller ones for less time. Turn it out and rap the bottom, listening for a hollow sound. If in any doubt, return to the oven for 5 even 10 minutes more, either in the tin or naked.

It is better to err on the side of too much baking than not enough and disappointing to cut what appears to be a baked loaf only to find the texture gluggy, and this especially applies to wholemeal.

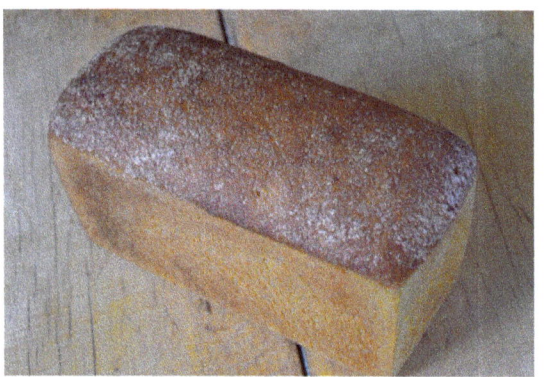

11. Make sure you place the baked hot loaf on to a wire cooling rack and leave it to cool thoroughly before cutting. Best to give it 8 hours to cool and cure.

The Sourdough Loaf

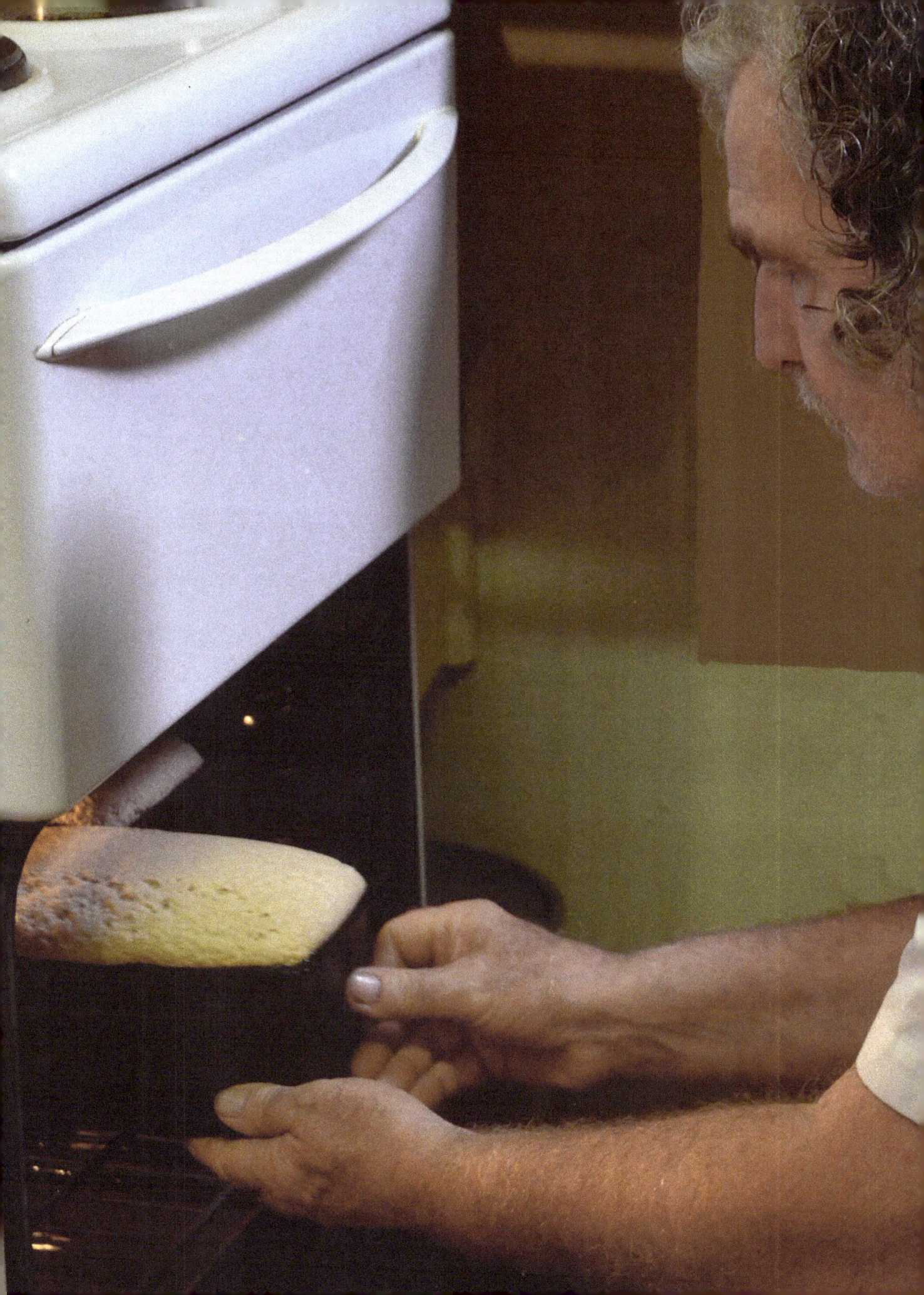

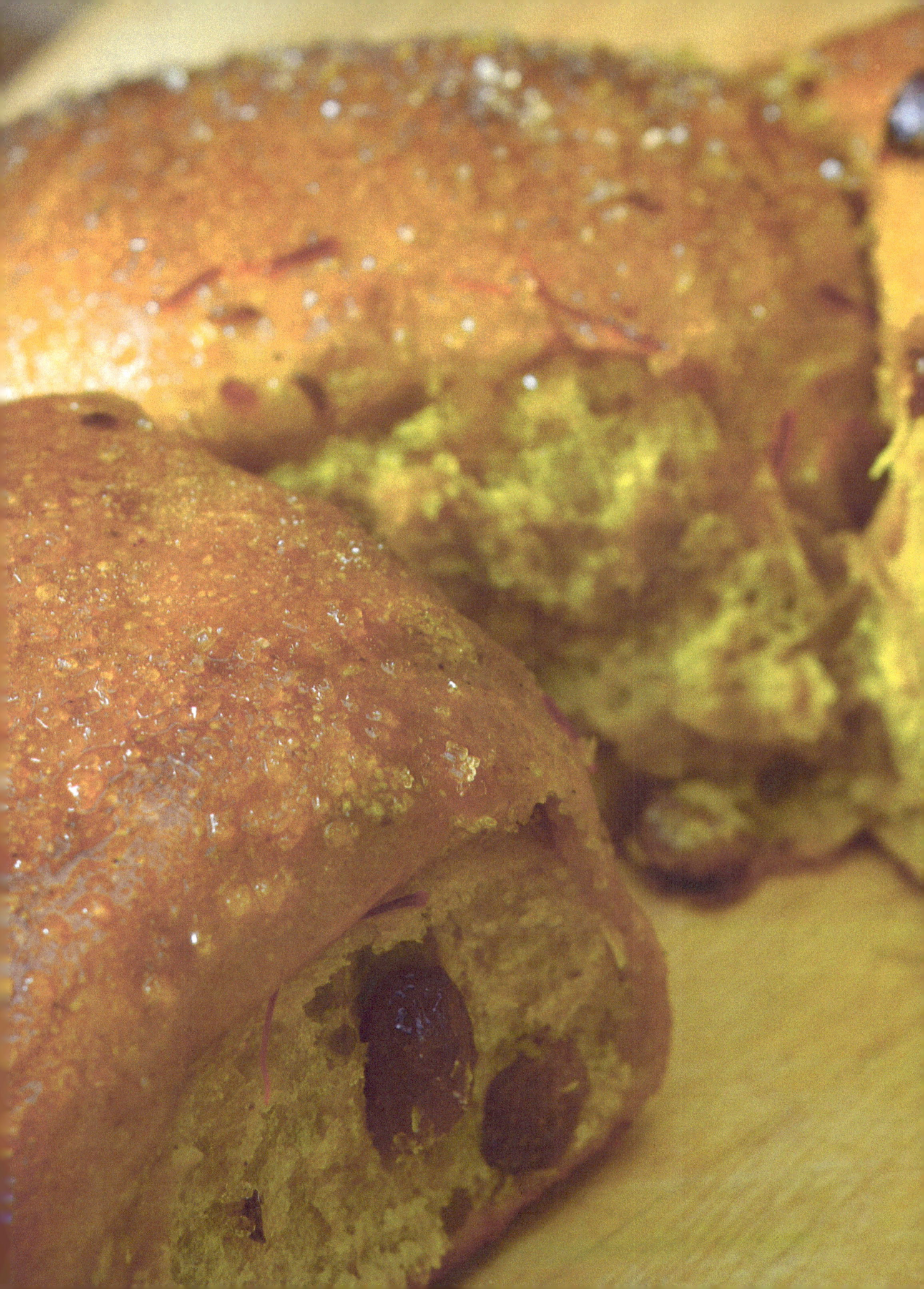

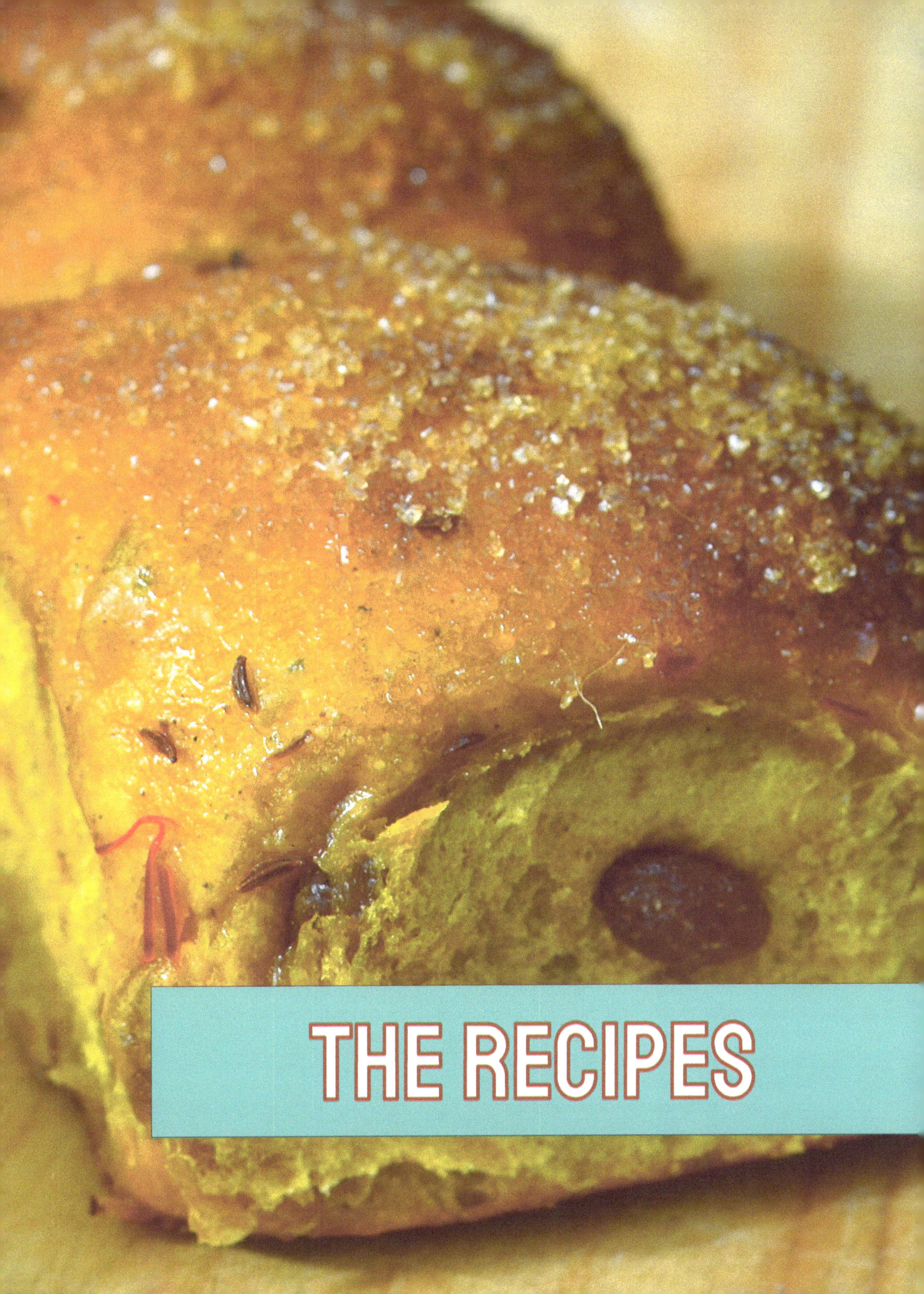

THE RECIPES

CRUSTY WHITE SOURDOUGH
The holey grail, bread zeppelin.

Ingredients.

- 500 g white flour, preferably organic, preferably bread flour.
- 250 g leaven, either wholemeal, brown or white.
- 280-300 g warm water about 27°C.
- 10 g sea salt.

There are three great versions of this bread. The wholemeal leaven gives a more coloured loaf, nicely flecked with golden bran and germ. The brown, or sifted flour leaven, is very flavoursome and smooth, my choice for an outstanding bread, and what I used in the original "casalinga", white torpedo-shaped crusty sourdough. Using the white leaven gives the whitest lightest bread, is less grain-flavoured, but about the best white bread there is.

I am much indebted to Nick and Maria, a Sicilian couple who had a grocery store adjacent to my first Melbourne bakery. Maria kept us alive with home-made Sicilian food. She was initially intrigued to learn we had a shop nearby and were baking in a wood-fired oven.

I took her a few loaves which she inspected and said they were "o-k", careful not to look me in the eye. It wasn't until I took the first good crusty white that a huge Sicilian smile awoke on a generous face framed with such black hair. "What would you call it?" I asked. "Oh it's a casalinga", Nick insisted as though curious we didn't know what the commonest item of food was called. The name stuck and it wasn't until many years later, a speaker of a more northern Italian tongue opined to me eyes heavenward that "casalinga" was "Sicilian (meridionale) slang".

Method
Follow the crusty bread method (pp 81 - 84) for baking instructions for this traditional loaf.
The quantities make one large loaf, or a small loaf and flatbreads, pizza bases or to use as a pre-ferment for buns and bakery sweets.

This recipe produces a soft slightly sticky dough, depending on how much water you add and how game you are. Using 270g of water gives an easy handleable loaf which will have a regular texture. Using 300g of water will give a very soft sticky dough, making a holey, soft but crusty bread. This sort of dough isn't easy to handle, but it is do-able, especially using the bakers slip as one of your hands.

To accentuate the holey structure, if you have the time and interest, fold this dough over itself a few times gently every half hour during its initial proof.

If using a white leaven, make sure it is at an advanced stage of frothy readiness. Wholemeal and brown leavens are easy to activate and are virtually always ready but white leaven can be slow to climax.

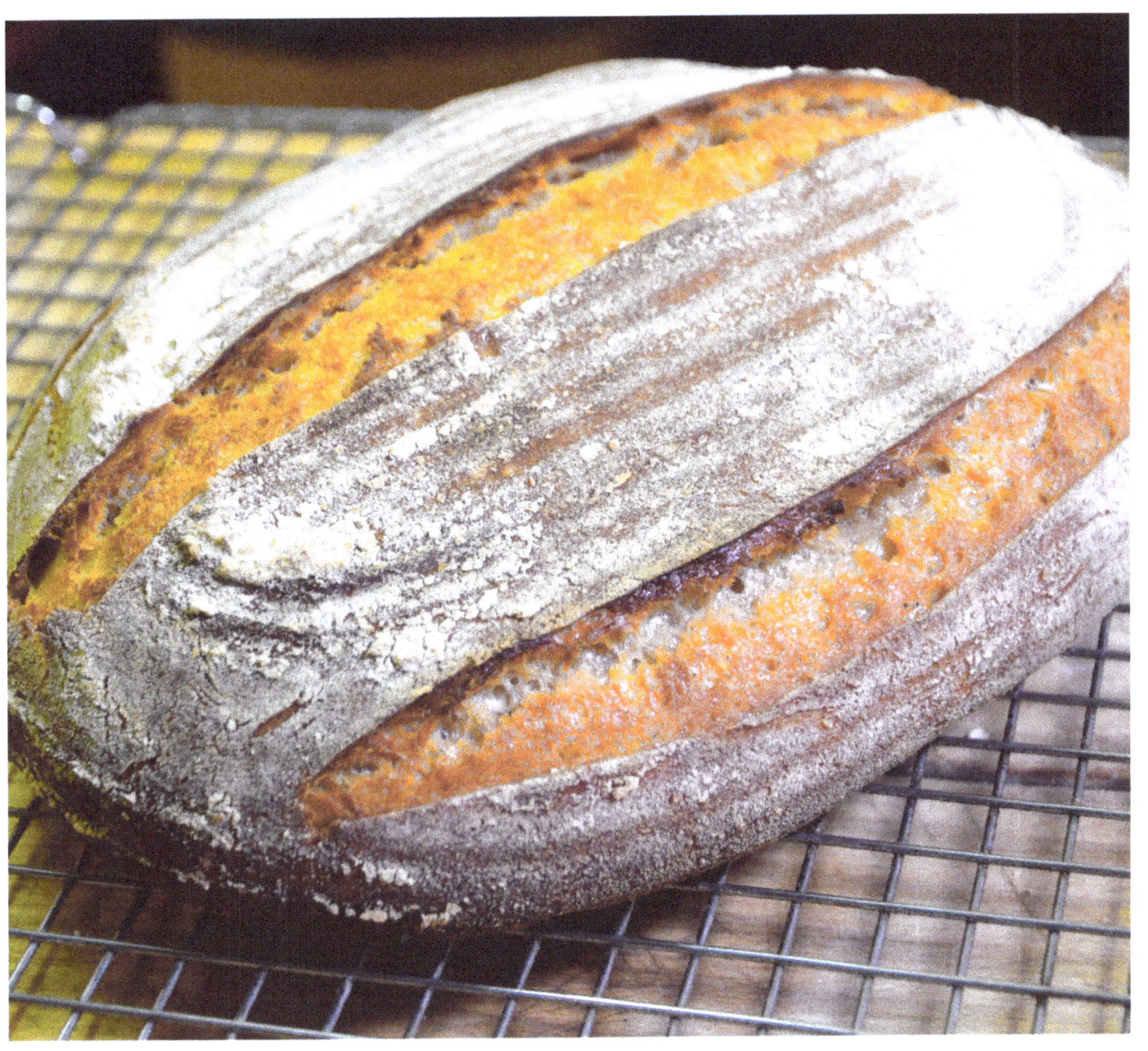

CRUSTY BROWN BREAD

Ingredients.

- 500 g sifted "light" wholemeal, flour.
- 250 g leaven from the same flour.
- 270 g warm water.
- 10 g sea salt.

After a good wholemeal, this is my favourite bread, and a historical favourite, being the most commonly made sourdough from antiquity, particularly in France and Belgium.

It is all in the flour really. Brown bread is made from a stoneground wholemeal which has been sifted to remove the coarse bran (see p 37)). This was the most common flour of the past as white flour, sifted through silk, was costly and not widely available. The flour retains germ and fine bran and is full of flavour, but lighter than a wholemeal.

Method

Follow the crusty bread method (pp 81 - 84) for baking instructions for this traditional loaf.

Because this flour ferments faster than a white, having more nutrients, the first proof should be for just one hour.

Brown bread (called a "crusty country" in my Melbourne bakeries) is perfect, and a tradition. Risen in a round basket and then slashed with a cross (to let the devil out) or the complete square cross-cut (hash tag).

Add an extra 10g of water to make this a really good tinned loaf.

Roll in sesame seeds or other seeds if desired.

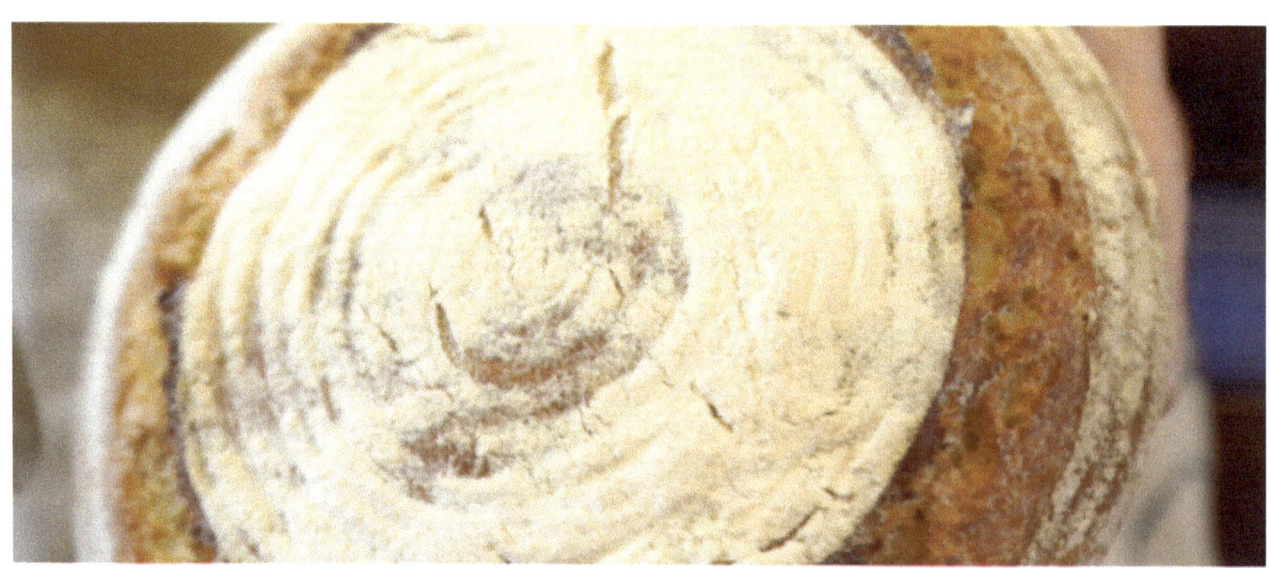

The Sourdough Loaf

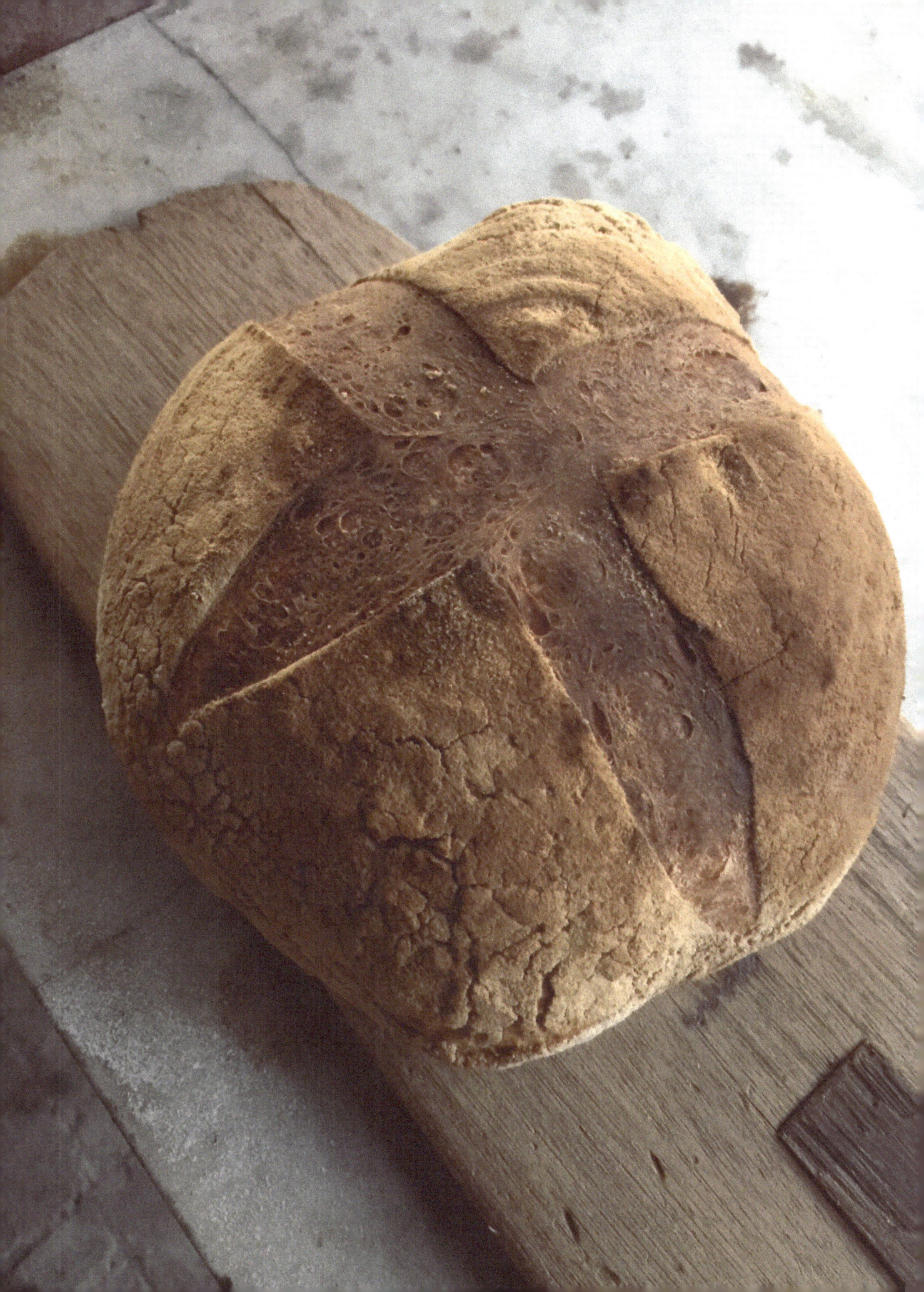

BOULE

Ingredients.

For 2 loaves of 2kg each:

- 2 kg sifted wholemeal flour.
- 1 kg leaven from the same flour.
- 1.15 kg warm water.
- 30 g sea salt.

This recipe is for big 3kg rounds (boule), once common in Europe. If you have the facilities, these are well worth making as the size somehow improves the loaf, and if baked in a woodfired oven, you will never make any other bread. I mention this, because some of you will have a wood-fired "pizza" oven and this is a great adventure.

Method

Follow the crusty bread method (pp 81 - 84) for baking instructions.

The recipe is for 2 loaves at 2kg each. Graduate to 2 loaves at 3kg by increasing the recipe by 1/3.

To prove/rise this bread, use anything of correct size, such as a cloth-lined large bowl, or the large plastic strainers common in Asian food stores, with a cloth or canvas lining. You will need an extra-wide peel, "the bat", to load these into an oven.

Bake for 45 minutes to an hour in mellow heat on the stones of a woodfired oven.

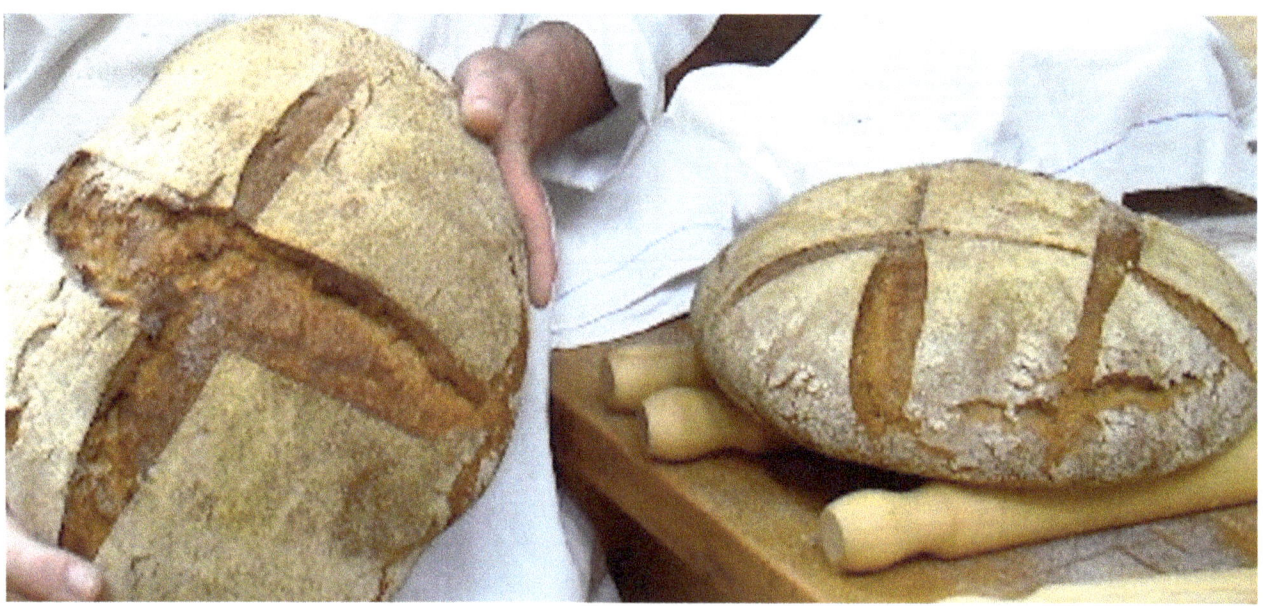

The Sourdough Loaf

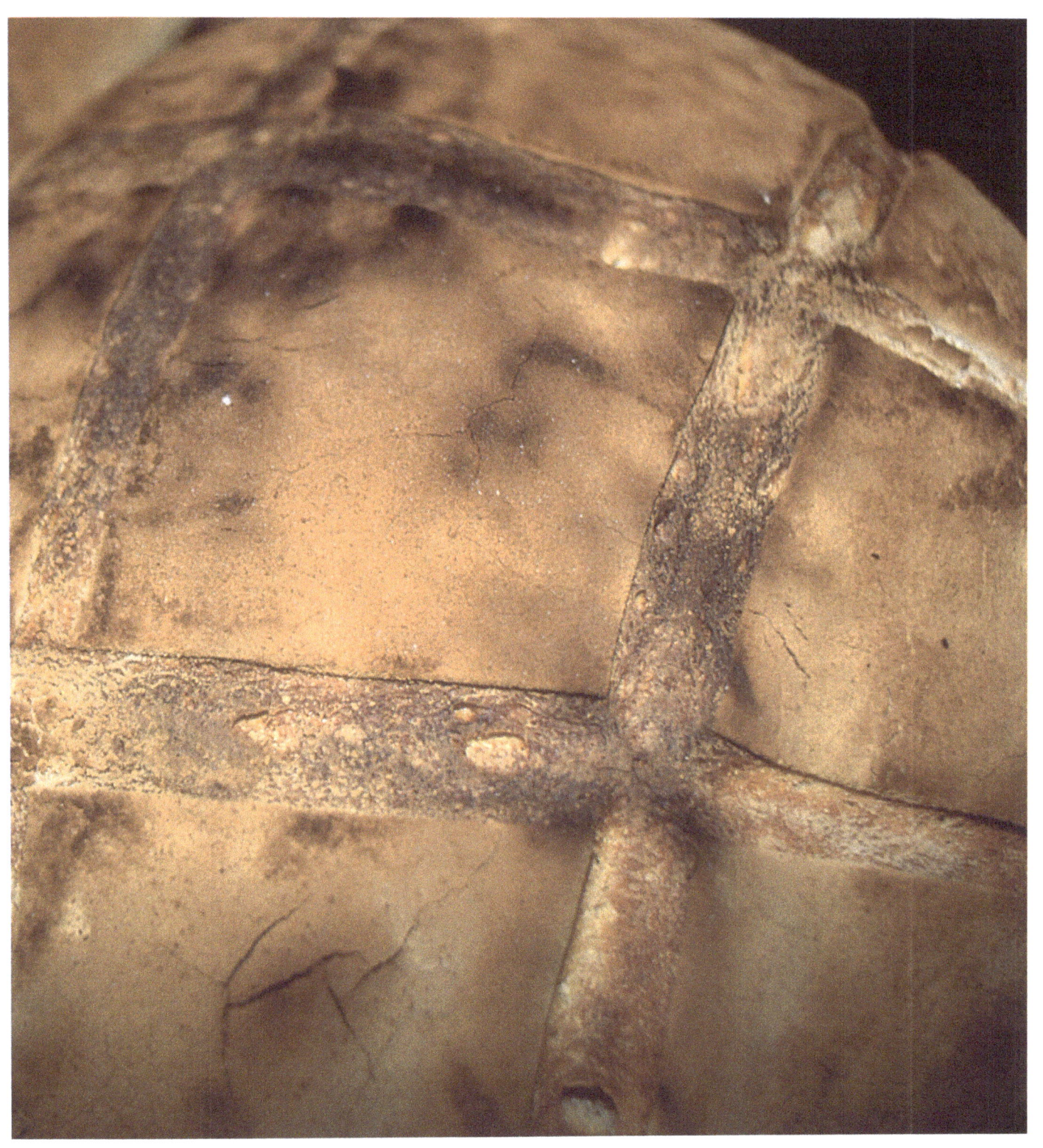

The Sourdough Loaf

PANES CUM TOTO

"Bread with all (the total)" Wholemeal wheat bread.

Ingredients.

- 1 kg organic stone-ground wholemeal wheat flour.
- 500 g wholemeal leaven.
- 670 g warm water (25°C).
- 20 g sea salt.

This is the bread by which all others are measured, the tastiest, the most wholesome, the essence of the "wholegrain". Called pane integrale in Italian and pain complete in French, says it all, with "integrale" meaning "integral" or "complete", and complete meaning, well, complete - in every way.

My local supermarket is advertising a fully white factory bread, "with the fibre of wholemeal in disguise" in which the fibre is "hidden" so children especially can have their cake and eat it as well! It's a pity wholemeal bread is seen as a penance.

The apparent demonisation of wholemeal as "brown" and "dark", and the triumphal ascendancy, supremacy, of white bread may have semiotic roots we would prefer to ignore. Can supremacy of the white be based on flavour and texture. - or any rational let alone gastronomic parameter?

Few people have actually tasted a proper wholemeal bread, as the supermarket ones are simply dyed brown and it is a rarity to find a good wholemeal, even in a groovy organic bakery. This wholemeal bread is not at all "heavy", as poorly-made wholemeal can be. Well-made and baked, it is light on the digestion and "eats well".

By gastronomic standards, which include organoleptic as well as cultural markers, sourdough wholemeal bread is a significant benchmark which embodies agriculture, displays skill, quality, and the elements of flavour ... what is there not to like?

Any food eaten with this wholemeal is elevated to greatness because far from being intrusive or overwhelming, the flavour of properly made wholemeal melds with other flavours, especially good cheese, enhancing them and extending them into the truly delicious.

As mentioned, different flours will produce different results, especially with stone-ground wholemeals. I remember reading Elisabeth David's account of making bread with superb-tasting soft Irish wholemeal, and being struck by the difference to my medium strength Australian wholemeal. Her method would have produced an unsatisfactory bread with my flour and if used on

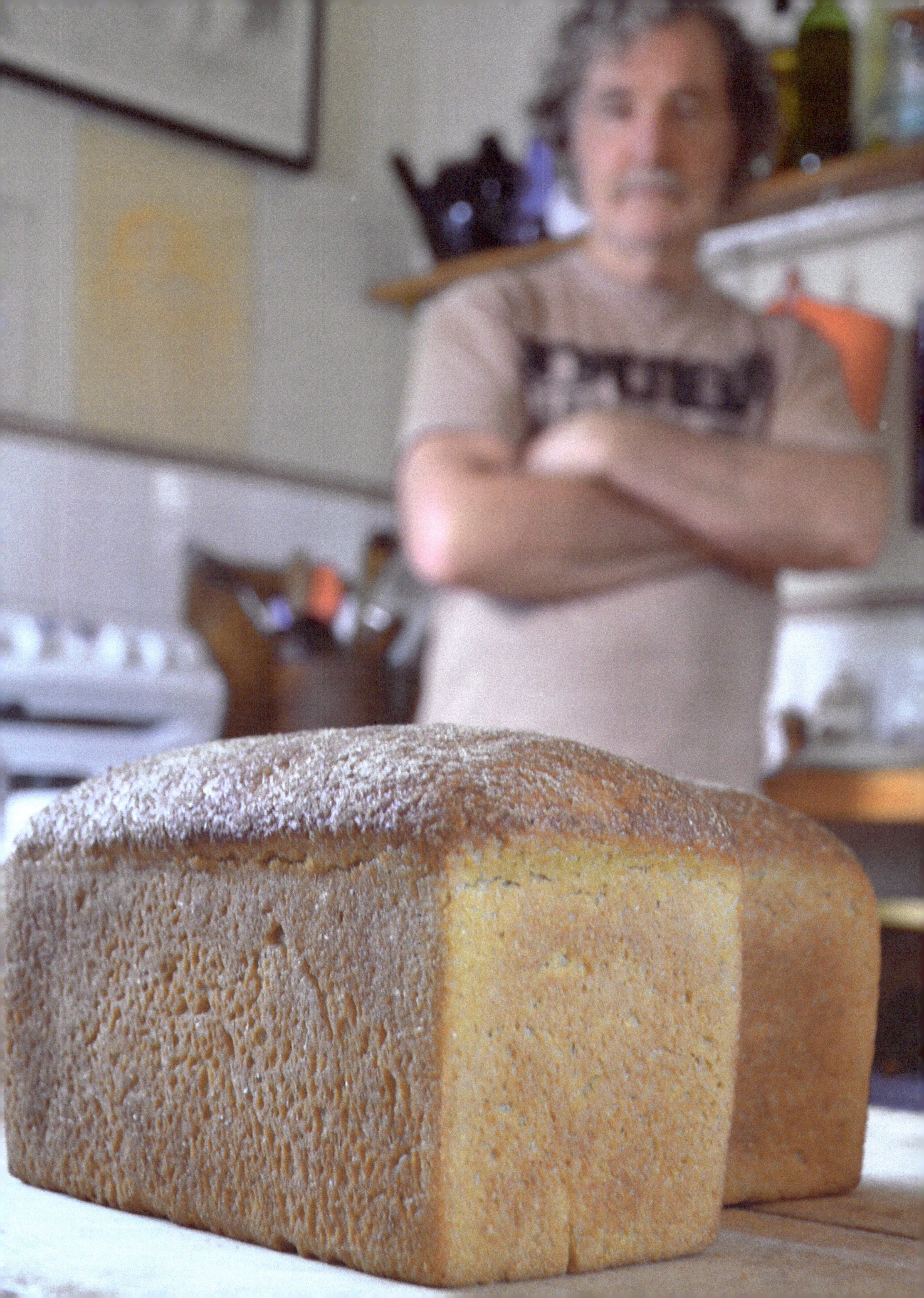

a strong Canadian wholemeal, a similarly bad result, yet the method she employed was entirely correct for the sweet soft Irish flour.

Follow either the crusty bread method (pp 81 - 84) or if baking as a tin bread, use the tin bread method (pp 85 - 87) for this bread.

Toasted, buttered with sweet butter and eaten with fresh oysters, sourdough wholemeal is a traditional and ancient treat from the 'before time' worthy of the now.

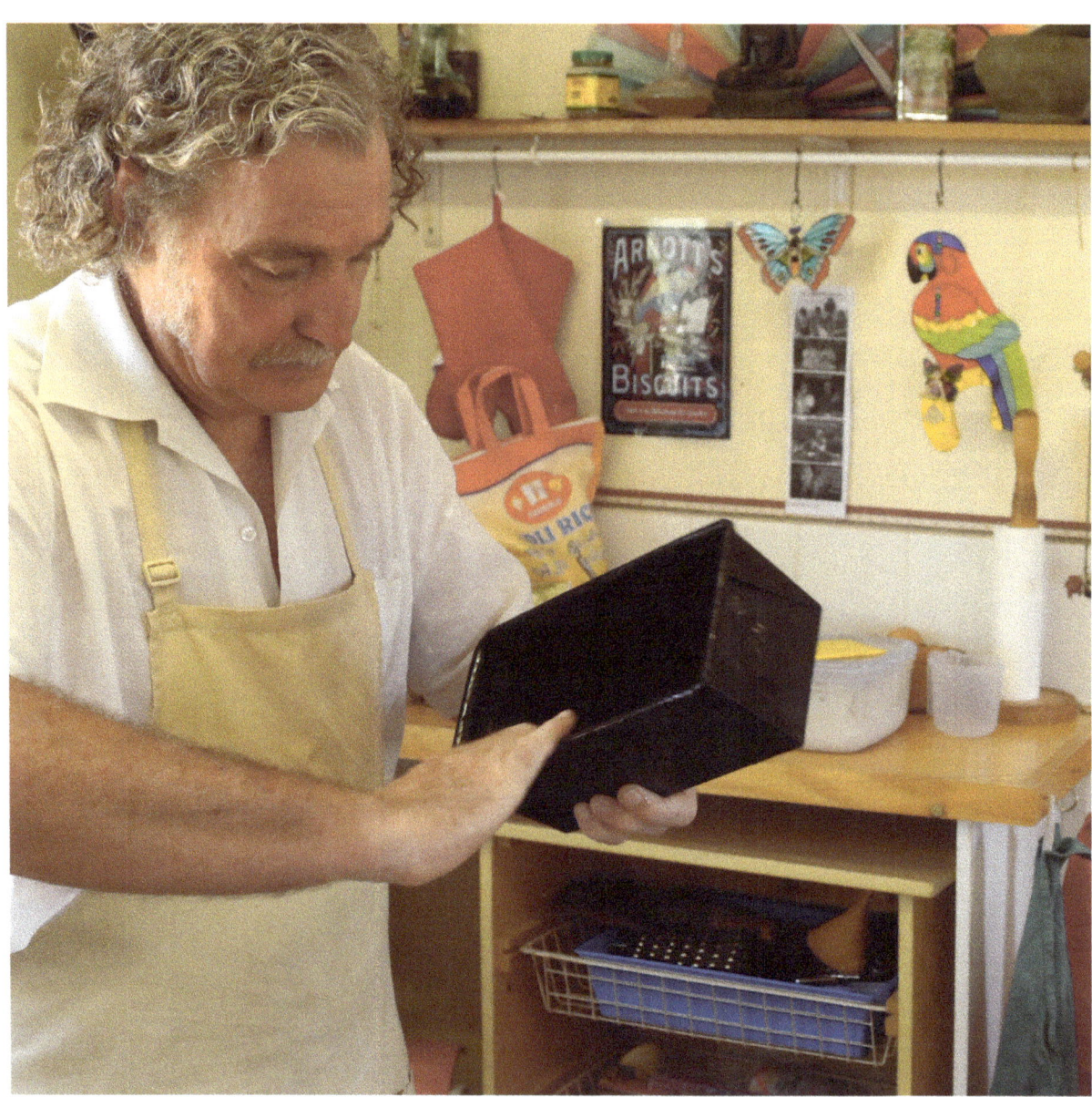

The Sourdough Loaf

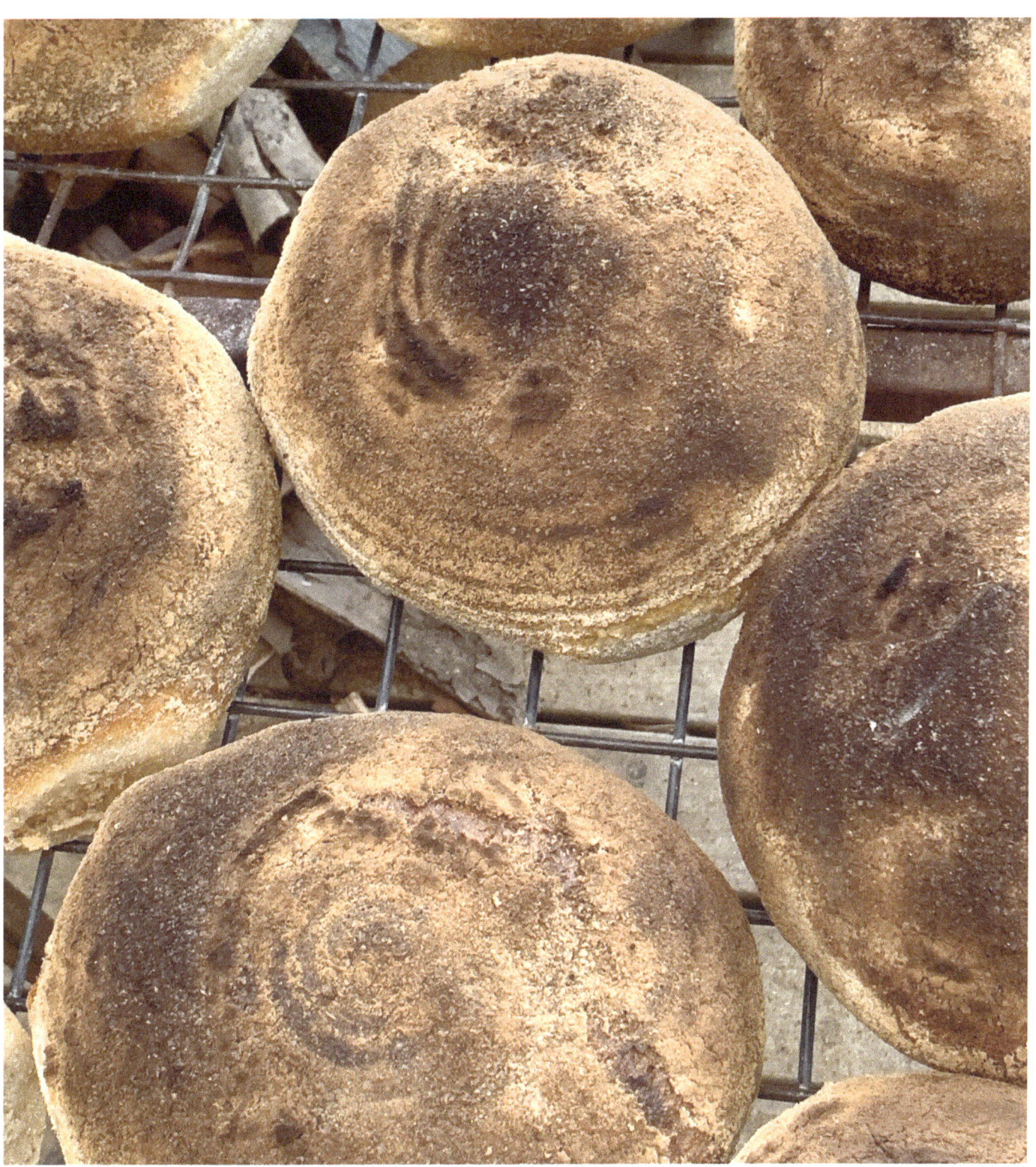

CRUSTY CHICKPEA BREAD

Pane con ceci.

Ingredients.

The leaven:

- 100 g chickpea flour.
- 120 g water.
- Pinch of sea salt.
- 2 tbsp of the stock leaven.

The bread:

- 550 g strong white bread flour.
- 220 g chickpea leaven.
- 230-250g warm water.
- 10 g salt.

This is an enhanced protein bread. The crumb of this bread has an attractive yellowish tint, with superb flavour from the fermented chickpeas. Chickpea flour is "raw" and "beany" tasting unless cooked or fermented. Leavens with chickpea flour need a pinch of salt or they go "off", but regular leaven does not need salt at all.

The fermentation of Pane con ceci is significant in that the considerable amount of protein they contain is de-complexed and meshes perfectly with wheat protein to create even more available protein. Nutty chickpea flavours and "pappadam" aromas are also released as the ferment "cooks" the chickpeas (in archaic terms), creating miso-like and cheesy flavours, which make this bread "scrumptious" according to some. Toasted (bruschetta), rubbed with garlic and spread with good butter or extra-virgin olive oil, this bread is a triumph.

Method

The night before, or about 12 hours before starting, make a leaven with the chickpea flour and your "stock" leaven. Cover and keep warm. This will be active after 8 hours. It separates, so stir well and leave another 3 hours to re-activate and "dome" up.

Mix the leaven into the warm water and whisk. Add the flour and salt, mix well and knead for a few minutes until smooth.

Cover, keep warm and proof for 2 hours. Reshape it, round the dough and rest for 2 minutes. Roll into a shape to fit your basket/banneton, dredge with flour (a mix of white and chick pea flours) and place in the basket. Cover and keep warm for 2 - 2 ½ hours further until well-risen.

Pre-heat the oven to 250°C, turn the loaf out onto a hot tray, slash it , place in the oven, turn the heat down to 200°C and bake for 25 minutes.

Alternatively, bake it in a tin for 35-40 minutes at 200°C.

CRUSTY CHESTNUT BREAD

Pane con castagne.

Ingredients.

The leaven:
- 100 g chestnut flour.
- 120 g water.
- 2 tbsp of stock leaven.

The bread:
- 550 g strong white bread flour.
- 220 g chestnut leaven.
- 230-250 g warm water.
- 10 g salt.

Make a leaven with chestnut flour in the same way as the chickpea leaven, but no need for salt. Proceed as with pane con ceci.

This makes an outstanding sweet-tinged loaf with the aroma of roasted chestnuts wafting from the auburn crust.

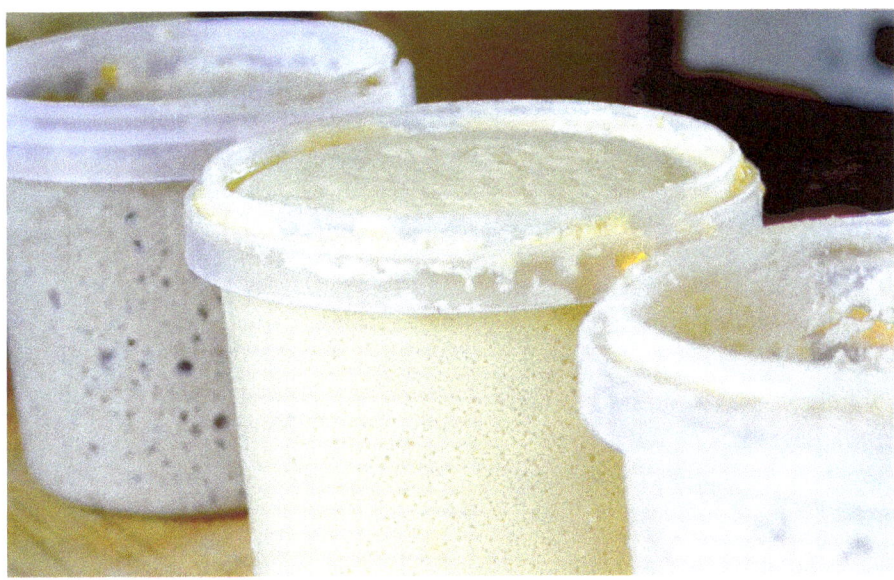

GREAT WHITE

Sandwich bread.

Ingredients.

- 400 g strong white bread flour.
- 200 g leaven, wholemeal or white.
- 220 g warm water (27°C).
- 8 g sea salt.

This loaf is ideal for sandwiches and for fitting in to lunch boxes - and the toaster. Double the recipe if need be, it is always good to have one frozen, or perhaps both will be scoffed within days by hungry hordes.

Method
Follow the tin bread baking method (pp 85 - 87) and refer to Panes cum toto for this bread. Reduce baking time to 30 - 40 minutes at 200°C .

Warm the flour first if the weather is cold. This bread requires 2 hours initial proof, after which, and before tinning, give it a good knead to distribute gases evenly, because this is not a holey sourdough, we are after a more regular texture. Thorough re-kneading will distribute the trapped gases more evenly.

Place the finally shaped loaf into a well-oiled tin which should be warmed first. Put into its warm nest, covered with the tea-towel and plastic.
Be patient as this loaf usually rises slowly, and in any case, needs to fully rise. If the un-risen dough half fills the tin, be patient - it should rise to the very top. A few tiny holes will break the surface when the loaf reaches full proof. If in doubt, wait, but 2 ½ hours should be enough.

If the loaf isn't fully risen it will crack or form open seams due to excessive oven spring.

When the loaf is turned out onto the cooling rack, allow to cool for half an hour, then wrap loosely in a cotton tea-towel until fully cooled. This will make the loaf softer for those who like less-tough bread -"the seekers after smooth things".

Adding fats or oils enriches the sandwich loaf and makes a softer texture. There are many options:

Use whole milk, substitute 50g in the water quantity, for example, 50g whole milk and 170g water. Similarly use almond milk, coconut milk, soymilk or other plant milk. Pureeing wholeseed sesame butter "tahina" with the water makes a delicious enriched soft loaf. Pureed tofu is also an excellent addition, boosting protein and "improving" the texture. Add 3 tablespoons to the dough.

Adding 1 tablespoon of extra-virgin olive oil or a cold pressed nut or seed oil, or pure cream to the dough will also make a softer crumb.

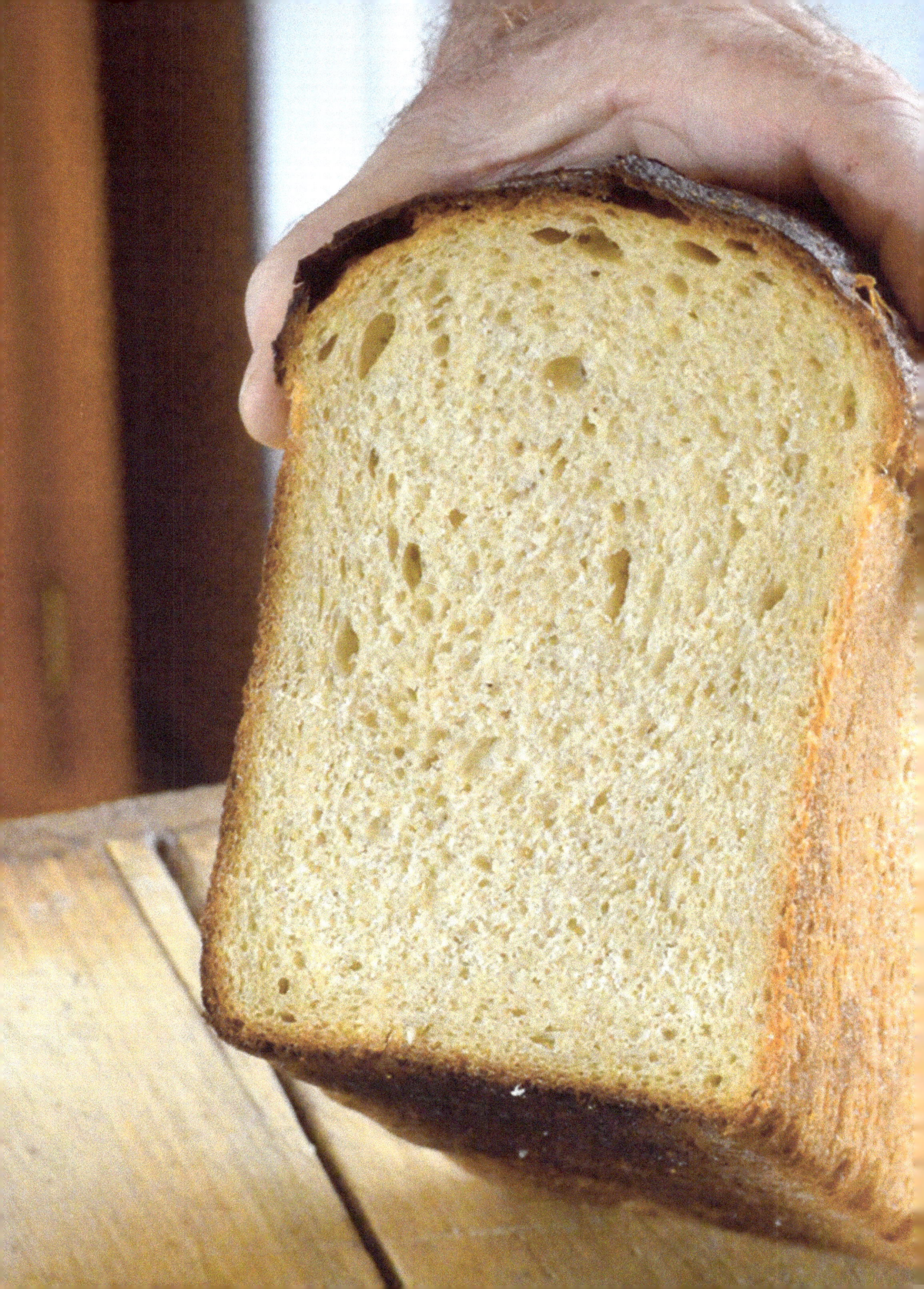

CORN BREAD

Ingredients.
- 150 - 180 g of boiling water.
- 120 g coarse yellow corn meal.
- Pinch of sea salt.
- 500 g crusty white or crusty brown dough.
- 100 g extra flour, white or sifted wholemeal.

This makes about the best toast, and invites many excellent toppings: spicey kidney beans, roasted pumpkin, avocado ...

I always bake this in smallish round tins, so the bread domes nicely. Rolled in coarse cornmeal, it is a very attractive and popular bread.

Choose coarse cornmeal for this bread. If the only meal available is fine, reduce the water to 150g.

Make the corn bread with the remnant dough of any of the white, brown, wholemeal or rye recipes. The dough must have had an initial proof first.

Method
The very first step is to add the boiling water to the coarse yellow corn meal. Add a good pinch of sea salt, stir it well and set aside for one hour. The cornmeal will soften and swell.

After the cornmeal has soaked, add the dough and add 100 g of extra flour.

Chop the dough into pieces, and mix in the cornmeal mixture and the extra flour until well incorporated. Knead briefly to form a smooth dough.

Cover and keep warm, proof for 1 hour.

Gently reshape the dough with a few folds, form the final shape, either a round or oblong, and roll in coarse cornmeal. Place in a pre-warmed tin, or floured basket if you want a crusty bread. Cover and keep warm for an hour or hour and a half, until well-risen. It should double in bulk. Pre-heat oven to 200°C.

Bake for 30 minutes for a tinned version.

If making a crusty shape, the oven should be pre-heated to 250°C then reduced to 200°C as the loaf goes in. Turn it onto a pre-heated baking tray, slash it once or twice and bake for 20-25 minutes.

This recipe makes outstanding flatbreads which are easy and fuss-free, and well worth trying.

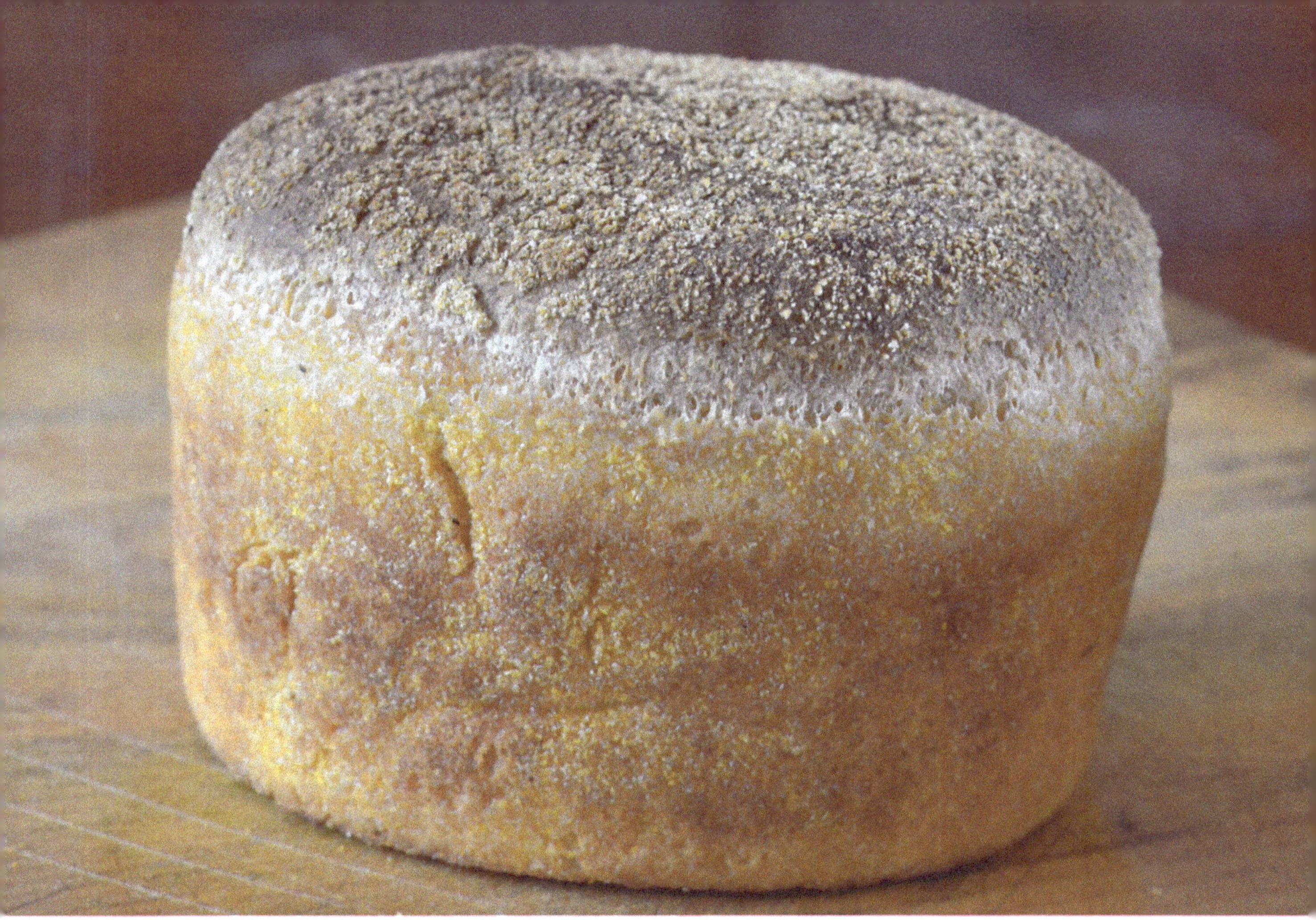

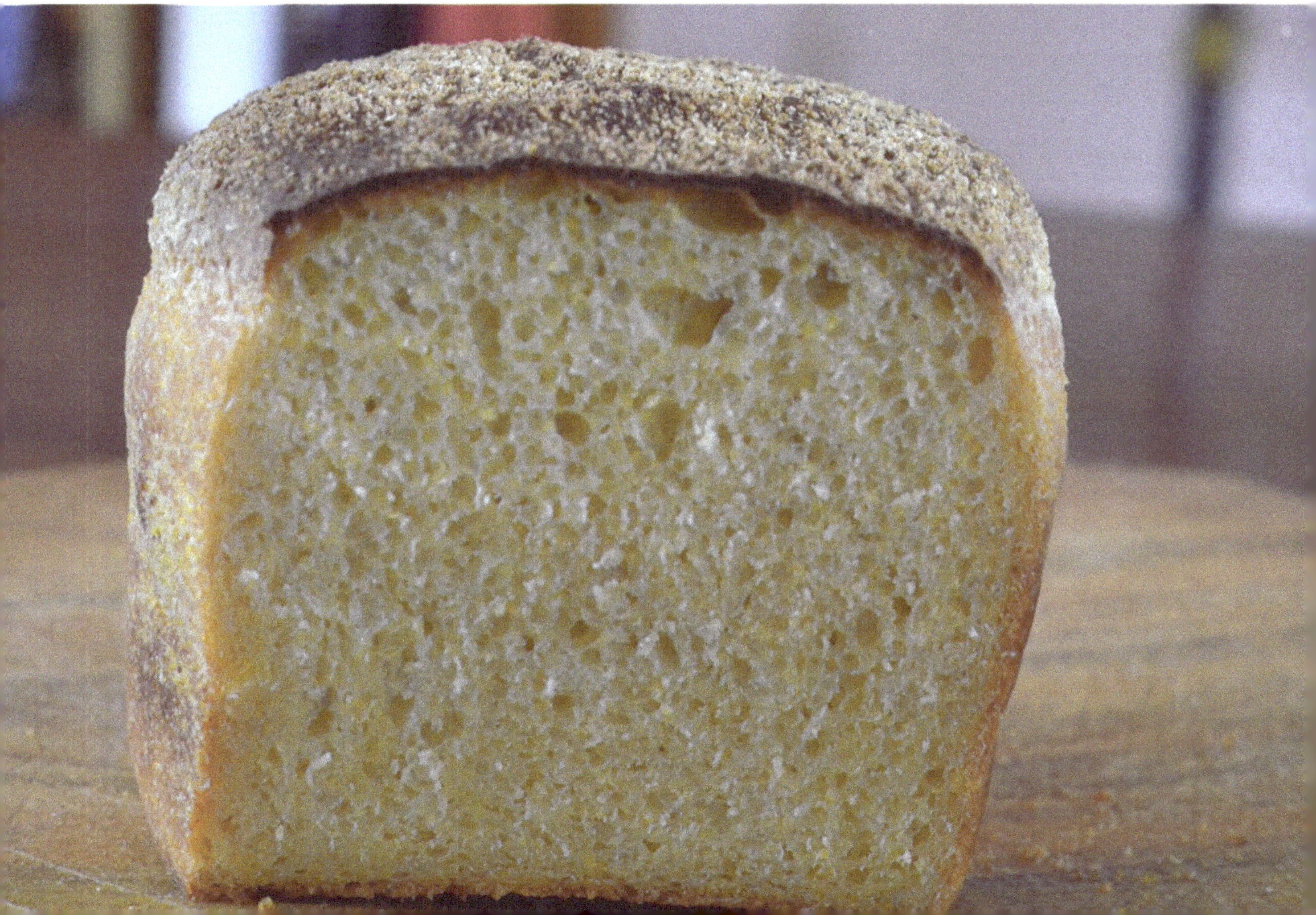

OTHER "CORN" BREADS

"Corn" is the archaic term for any cereal. When Europeans first came into contact with the American grain, they simply called it "corn" as was their habit, and the name stuck. It is of course, Maize.

The corn bread recipe is a useful template for making breads from other types of "corn" cereals. The polenta can be substituted with millet meal, barley meal, quinoa, amaranth, teff, brown rice or sorghum meal, all of which should be a fraction more "gritty" than a flour. Besides soaking, these meals can also be cooked to a thick porridge before adding to the dough, or made into a leaven.

If the meal is fine, as with the polenta, use less water as above.

Barley meal greatly benefits from being lightly toasted as is done in Tibet. This really accentuates the malty flavour and makes the grain more appetising. If you have a grinder, the best way is to toast the whole barley and then grind it. Otherwise, lightly toast it or any cereal meal in a pan on the stove top or in the oven.

Similarly quinoa and millet benefit from light toasting to eliminate any bitterness which is sometimes encountered with these grains. Often this is because the flour is old. If you have a grinder of any sort, for example a coffee grinder, make your own meals from the wholegrains, to ensure excellent flavour.

Add good unsalted butter or ghee to the barley bread for an even more delicious result. Simply warm the butter and add when the final dough is being made. Another flavoursome, nutritious addition to these grain breads is toasted tahina, or sesame butter. The best sesame butter is made from unhulled sesame seeds. Simply toast it gently in a skillet until it is aromatic with sesame-ness and grind it. Use one tablespoon per loaf.

The addition of good quality fats to grain breads tends to balance the inherent dryness and create a smooth texture with enhanced nutrition.

Other worthwhile additions to grain breads are nut and seed meals. These won't affect the dough consistency much, so experiment to create enhanced breads both nutritionally and for great flavour.

For example barley bread benefits from the addition of half of one cup of hazelnut meal per loaf. Lightly toast the hazelnuts first, then grind to a coarse or fine meal. This is a traditional practice in what used to be the barley-eating countries, and is historical for good reason, being very delicious.

Similarly, toast sunflower seeds and grind to add to quinoa and amaranth breads. All being Andean foods, the flavours have a "local" synergy.

Almond meal is a perfect addition to the corn bread recipe.

Hemp seed is a valuable food with about the best range of fats, besides really good flavour, and is worthwhile including in any of these breads, as are ground flax seeds.

Meals made from nuts and seeds, rather than whole seeds or chunks of nut, are used because they are eminently digestible. The tendency is to not chew so much, using meals enables better absorption of nutrients and also liberates the excellent flavours and aromas.

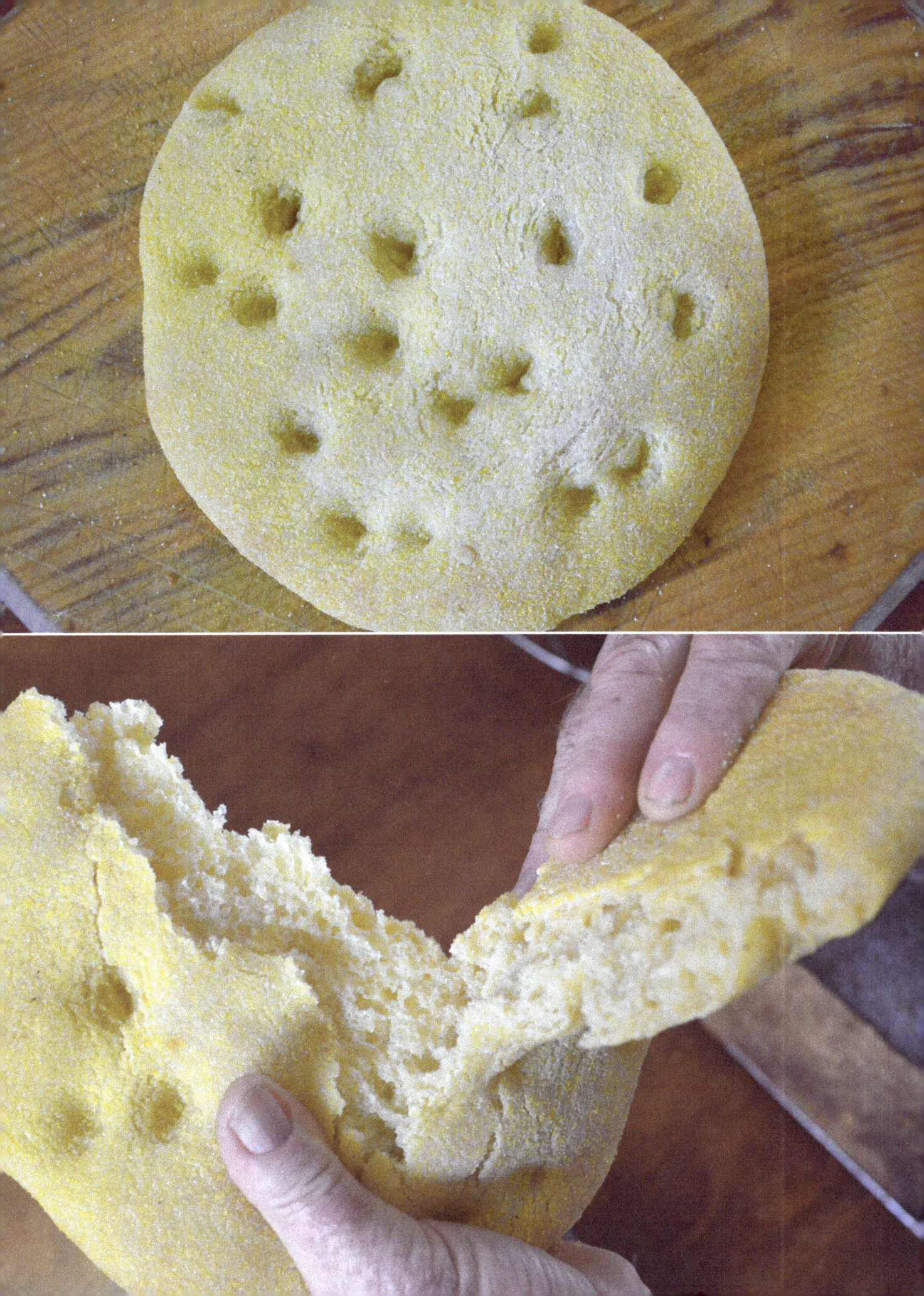

PAIN DE CAMPAGNE
Yeoman's Loaf.

Ingredients.

- 200 g sifted wheat flour.
- 200 g sifted "white" spelt flour.
- 100 g wholemeal rye flour.
- 250 g sifted wheat flour leaven.
- 270 g warm water.
- 10 g salt.

"Country bread" in French and as such is distinct from the white or white-ish loaves traditionally favoured by Parisians.

In the past it was a hefty loaf, the same as the English yeoman`s loaf, always about 3 kg, large dark and round. This can be a strong-tasting loaf, well-fermented and composed of wheat, rye and spelt and/or emmer, as wholemeals or sifted. Depending on the harvest it may contain less or more of each cereal, but wheat being less available, was often not in the grist, so the loaf may be rye based….but never white as is sometimes seen today….and may even contain ground acorns, field peas and nuts.

This is a loaf to experiment with. In my bakeries it was made with two thirds sifted wholemeal wheat flour and one third wholemeal rye flour, and as such was very popular and well flavoured.

Substitute 50g of chestnut, chickpea or emmer flour in the rye quantity for a more interesting and authentic flavour.

Double the recipe for a big crusty loaf.

Method
Follow the procedure for the white crusty loaf, except the first proof is for one hour only as this ferments rapidly. Final proof is for 2 hours. If you like a strong-tasting bread of yore, ferment for 2 hours initially.

As this dough ferments rapidly it will tend to be soft and spread. It may not need slashing, but if you do slash it, use very shallow slits. Traditionally it was cut with a large "square" cut now known as a "hash tag" # .

Such loaves were often "bashed" instead of slashed, the bakers thumb deeply indenting the centre like a navel. To do this, push your thumb into the centre of the loaf, almost to the bottom immediately before baking.

SCHWARZBROT

Black Bread.

Ingredients.

- 750 g wholemeal rye flour.
- 750 g wholemeal rye leaven.
- 325 g warm water.
- 10 g sea salt.

This makes 2 large loaves, or halve the recipe for a single loaf.

Black bread has to be another ancestral staple. Historically a lot more people ate rye than wheat, as it could stand the cold and grow in poorer soils, and mostly the wealthy monopolised wheat. Rye was a symbol of status and its dark (prince of darkness) colour a signifier of taint compared to the white yeast breads of the nobles (or Parisians). Surprisingly, rye turns up in archaeological digs in Jordan from about 7000 BCE.

The flavour is sharp, on the kind side of sour with an almighty taste of dark, dark rye. It is immensely satisfying to eat and of course accompanies all the foods more common in colder climates, especially good hard cheeses.

Rye is also best stoneground, and 100% wholemeal stoneground is required for black bread. It may also be sifted, as is wheat flour, and this "light" rye also makes a black bread. Rye ferments rapidly, but because it has no superstructure-forming gluten, it is never a high rise. It is dense and heavy, but really light on the digestion. Proper black bread can be kept for months and is usually at its best about a week after baking.

Sometimes black bread is tinged with caraway, cumin or even coriander seed. If you enjoy this combination, use a teaspoon or 2 of caraway seeds.

Method
Mix the leaven into the water, and whisk well. Add the flour and salt and probably start to despair! It really is a mess and cannot be kneaded. Mix it well with the wooden spoon and bakers slip. Mixing until the dough is clear of lumps.

Form it into an oblong-ish shape with the slip and roll in rye flour until well-covered. Put the dough into an oiled tin with any seams on the bottom, don't bother to smooth it out, cover with a damp cloth and plastic and walk away for 4 hours.

It will have surpisingly morphed into a risen loaf with the top showing advanced fermentation, seams and some terrain, all very attractively powdered with snow-like rye flour.

Bake at 180°C for an hour, un-tin and bake naked for a few minutes if you suspect it is a bit gluggy, or if you enjoy that gutsy rye crust. Turn onto a cooling wire rack and definitely do not cut it for 8 hours. In fact leave it as long as possible before cutting, day 3 after baking being just right as the bread cures to perfection. It should be sliced thinly.

CRUSTY SPELT BREAD

Ingredients.

- 500 g white spelt flour.
- 250 g white spelt leaven.
- 260-280 g warm water.
- 10 g sea salt.

Spelt grain has made a spectacular recovery from being a relic crop. It was once widely grown and eaten from India to Europe and is a variety of wheat.

This bread is made from what is termed, "white" spelt, which isn't white at all, although it appears so, but the dough is nicely speckled light brown with the peculiar purplish/plum blush of spelt. "White" spelt is rarely roller-milled, and usually, the "white" is simply sifted stoneground spelt, an ideal flour really.

Spelt is a soft wheat, having a low gluten content, but it is high in non-gluten water soluble proteins, which makes it very digestible. Being a soft wheat it makes tasty crusty breads with a crunchier crust than regular wheat with an excellent nutty-oaten aroma.

Spelt varies a lot, depending on where it was grown and specifying exact water quantities is difficult. Being "soft" it does not absorb as much water as regular, especially strong, wheat flour. The recipe also makes a worthy baguette if you prefer. The crust is the very best baguette crust.

Method

Follow the crusty bread method (pp 81 - 84) and either use a spelt leaven made from scratch, or make a spelt batter and add 2 tablespoons of your stock leaven. Leave 8 hours to ferment. When it is really active, stir it well and wait about 3 hours for it to recover volume.

This recipe, as all of them, can be pushed to your limit. Using 260g of water will give an easy to handle bread with a regular, close crumb structure. As you add more water, all becomes edgey, the dough softer, harder to handle and the bread holier than thou, with the crunchy crust. Using 280g of water will make a difficult to handle sticky/slippery dough, and holey, very crusty bread, which is a classic flavour and texture.

The bakers slip comes in handy here as it can act as your second hand, flipping and rolling the sticky dough...so it doesn't stick. Remember to keep your hand movements rapid. Knead and mix for 4-5 minutes until the dough has some integrity and holds together.

It is relatively easy to make a very soft dough, by using a smaller stainless bowl, say with a 26cm/10 inch diameter. The loaf can be made and proofed in this bowl, and as you are initially mixing and kneading the sticky version, the bowl almost acts like your second hand, and can be spun as you knead and lift the dough with the slip.

When the dough is made, keep it warm and proof for 2 hours. Then, using a little dusting flour, round it, give it a 2 minute rest, and then roll it into shape. Roll in flour and place in the basket or banneton for 2 hours of final proof.

When the dough is ready to be baked, if making the softer dough, it will be edgy, so tip it onto a pre-heated tray and straight into a hot 250°C oven then turn the oven down to 180°C. Bake 30 minutes for a rustic crusty bread.

No need to slash or cut the crust if making the softer version, it will spread and form attractive rivulets in the crust and roasty topography. A firmer dough may be slashed once or twice, not too much or it may spread and open the cuts too far.

Alternatively, reduce loaf weight to 800g and reserve the rest for a flatbread or meaningful pizza base.

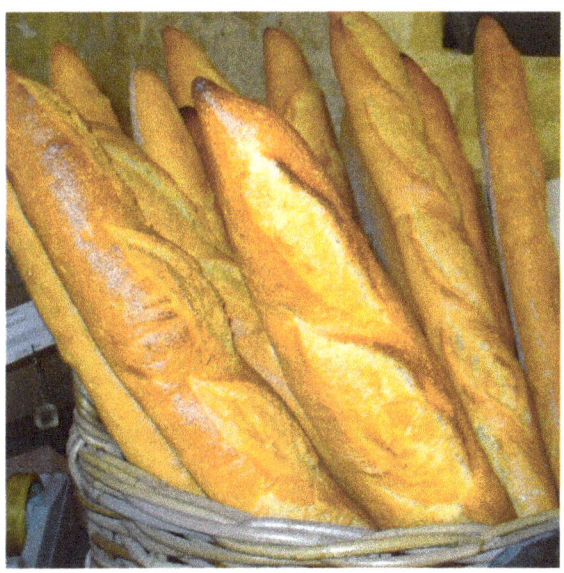

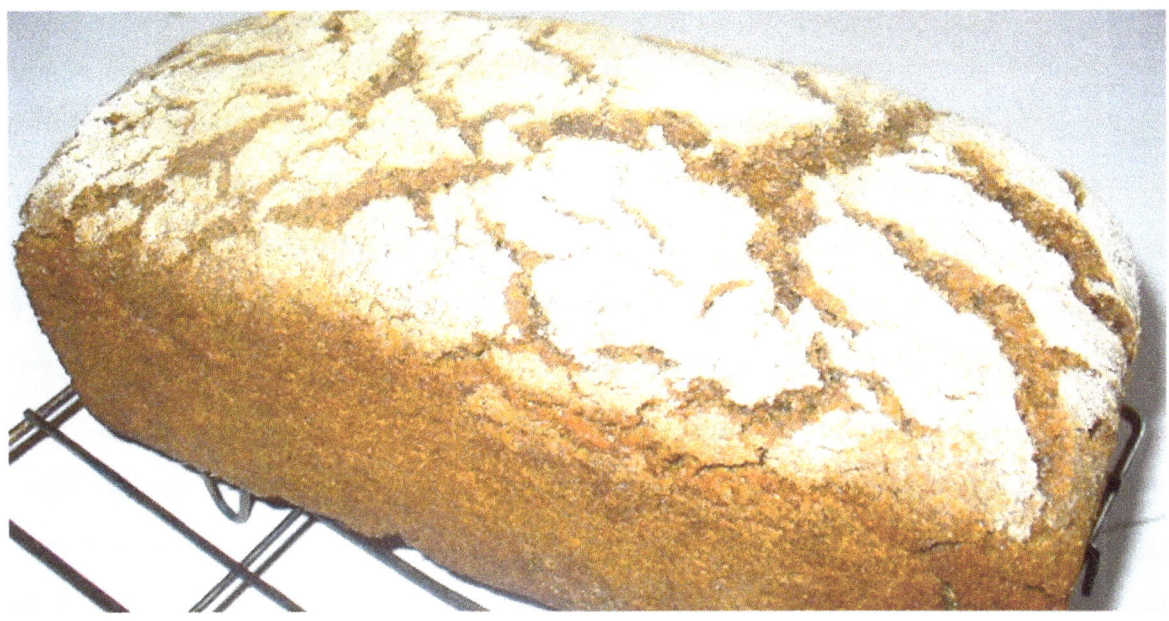

The Sourdough Loaf

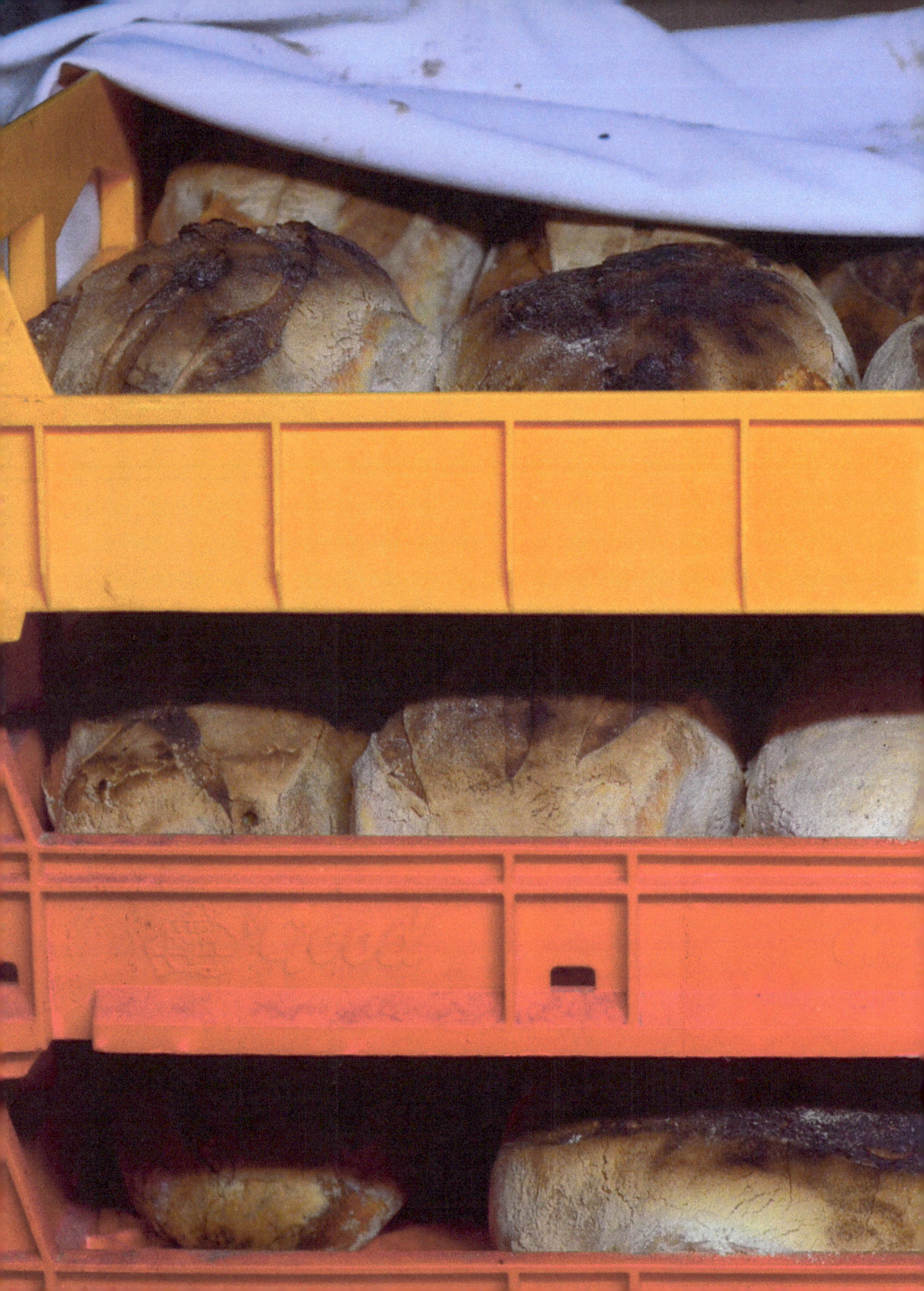

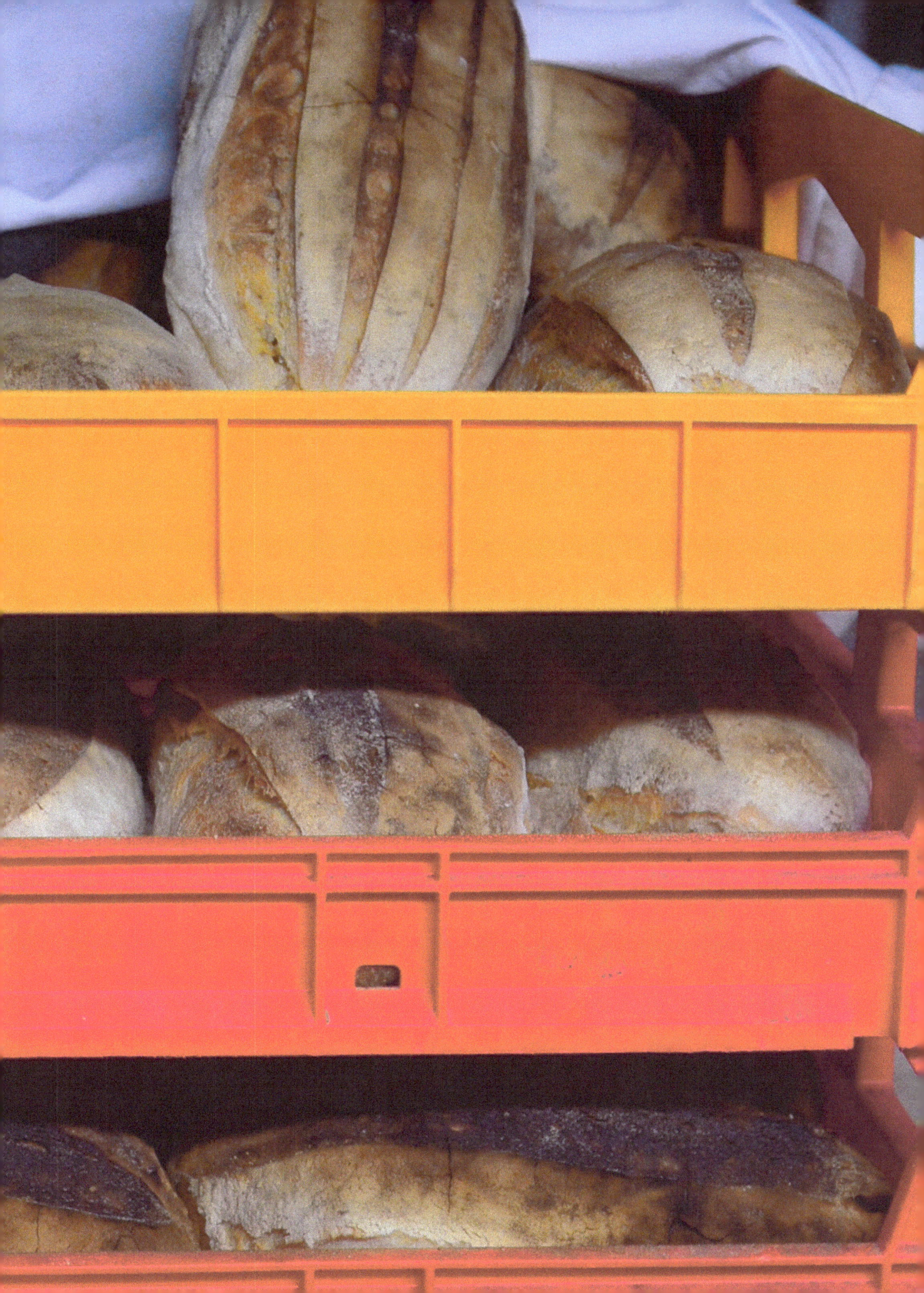

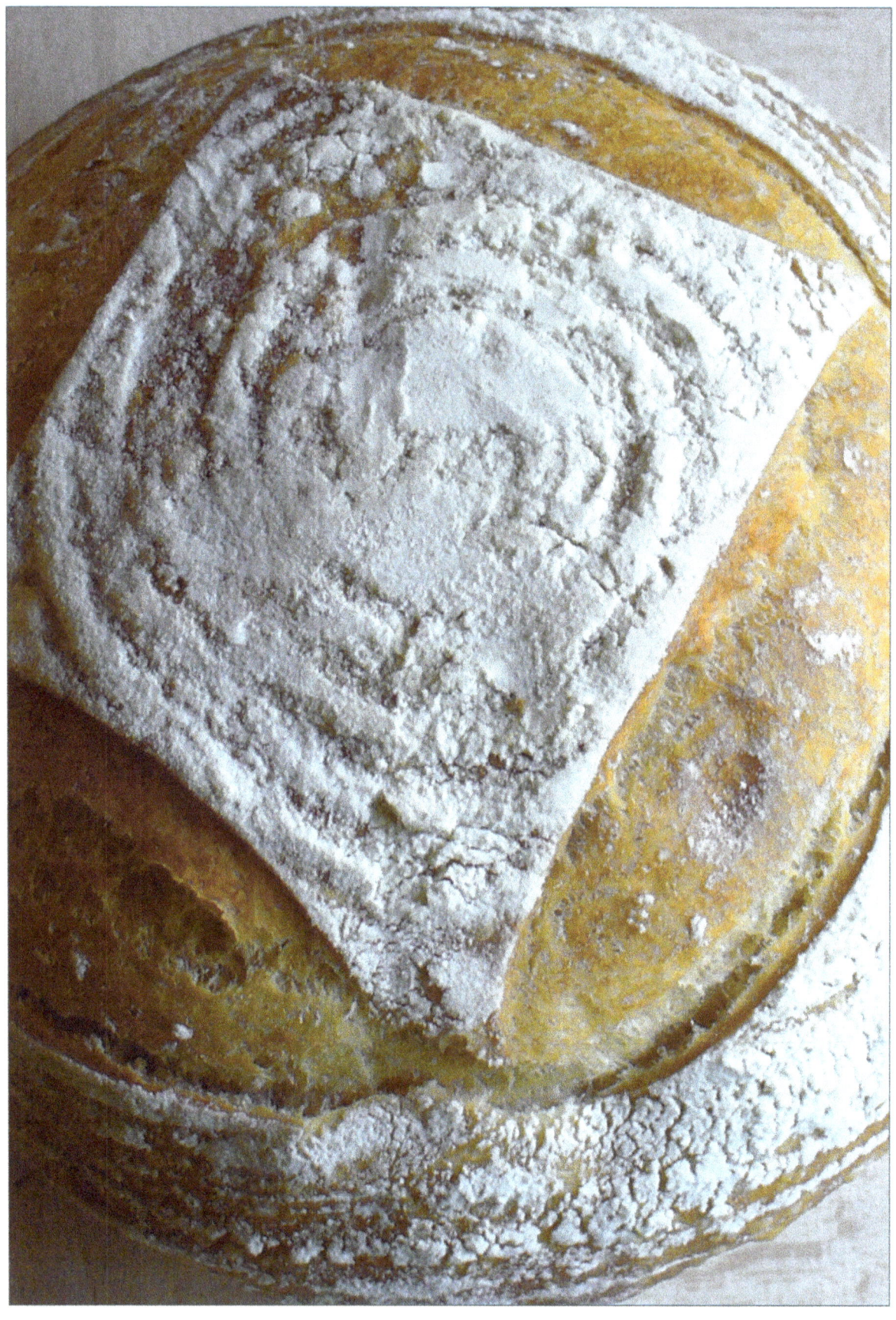

The Sourdough Loaf

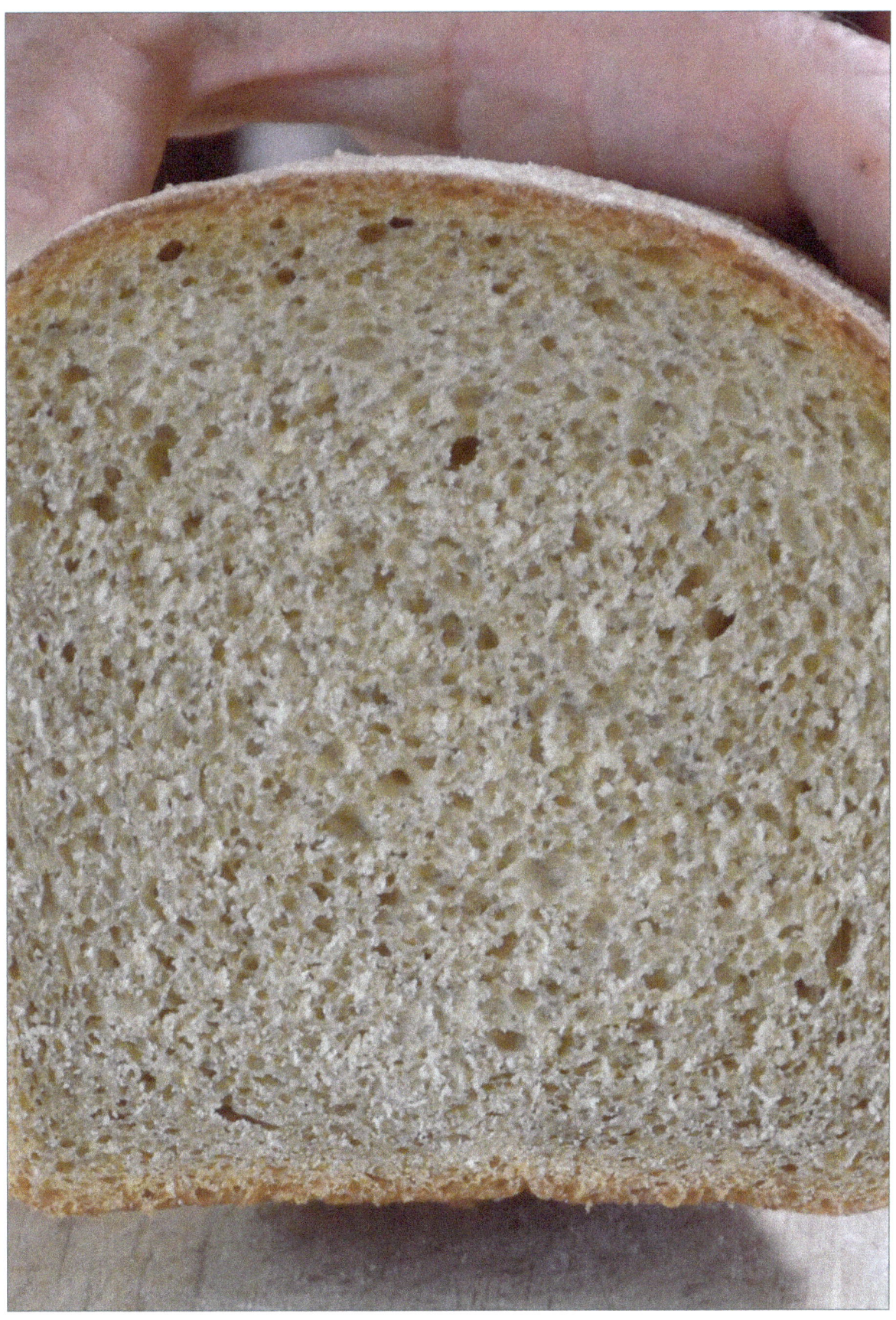

The Sourdough Loaf

EMMER BREAD

Ingredients.
- 410 g emmer flour.
- 350 g emmer leaven.
- 200 g warm water.
- 5 g salt.

Emmer wheat is the second oldest known wheat after einkorn. It was widely eaten as a wholegrain, a porridge (polenta) and in bread for 5000 years and more, being the staple of ancient Egypt and Rome. After a chance cross pollination of emmer with a wild grass, modern wheat was born, with a lot more genetic material as well and "new" proteins which seem to be allergenic to some and horsemen of the apocalypse to others.

Emmer flour is quite gritty and dry, with no soft white endosperm, and with virtually no extensible gluten, so it cannot form the steely geodesic structures of wheat doughs, instead something more like the nomadic yurt. With lower and less complex gluten than regular wheat, Emmer is easy to digest.

It ferments actively to produce a nice cakey crumb amid quite a soft holey texture. The trick is to de-programme the imprinting we carry about "bread", and make well-fermented flatbreads to enjoy instead of slices, which just could result in a culinary and gastronomic revelation.

If the slice beckons however, this bread can be made in a bread tin so the dough can ferment to its maximum and display that moist earthy crumb.

Emmer bread in ancient Egypt was baked in a conical clay pot which was sunk into a bed of coals. Another pot was up-ended on its rim sealing it like a miniature oven. This trapped the steam and encouraged the flinty emmer to soak up moisture. It also explains the puzzling conical things being carried to feasts depicted in ancient Egyptian frescoes. The resulting loaves were about 3kg in weight and perfectly conical. Only the geometry-prone ancient Egyptians would create bread as perfect cones! Granted this was ceremonial and not everyday bread, but 3kg cones of bread, wow! Surely this was a nose-cone replica of an interstellar vehicle!

The flavour of emmer is unlike regular wheat, being sweeter, more like an archetypical taste and aroma of "cereal", subliminally emotive, as finding the source of something atavistically nourishing and deeply delicious. Emmer bread has a similar unusual colour as einkorn with shades of lavender or purple, also seen in some heirloom wheat.

Emmer has been debunked as a relic and of interest only to the "rarity obsessed". It is however as relevant today as it was in ancient Egypt. It yields less than modern wheat per acre, but can be grown on marginal land, where wheat actually won't grow. It is also untainted by the sinister for-profit genetic meddling which has made modern wheat a problem child.

Nutritionally, emmer has a lot of protein, usually 15%, which is easily digested. Fermenting it unlocks the abundant minerals such as ancient plant sequesters, bestowing all the goodness we know through historical and cultural experience that are in whole cereal grains.

Method

As mentioned, emmer ferments rapidly and if a high ratio of leaven to flour is used, the bread is ready to bake in 2 ½ hours. The emmer leaven is robust. After 8 hours, it peaks and can then be stirred, "knocked-back", and will peak again more as a froth 3 hours later, when it is ideal to use.

If bread is then made using this leaven, it gives dramatic flavour and crust quality to the tawny loaf, demonstrating how emmer may be used creatively in modern baking.

This recipe for an emmer crusty bread or 2 flat breads is really quite fast. It is based on making the emmer leaven, which takes about 12 hours. I make the leaven in the evening, knock it back in the morning, and make bread in the afternoon. Making the leaven takes about 5 minutes in all.

Emmer dough benefits from a short-time kneading (2 minutes), as its gritty particles absorb the water. It does not form gluten strands but is quite a stable dough, and the kneading creates some integrity. It seems like gluten strands form, but they are ribbons not girders.

Mix all together with a strong wooden spoon, then use the slip and hands to fold and work it briefly and form into a coherent soft dough. Knead it briefly….or in a mixer on very low speed..

Cover and leave to prove for 1 hour. Turn it on to a lightly floured surface, fold it a few times, and form into a round. For an oblong basket, flatten the round and fold it on itself, roll it up like a pipe. Roll in emmer flour and place in the basket with the seam uppermost. Otherwise, roll the ball in flour and place in a round basket. Cover with a cloth and plastic and proof for 2 hours.

An option is to form the dough into a ball and sit it on a baking tray covered with a large bowl, as the loaf will spread, or brush the surface well with a good extra-virgin oil to prevent a hard crust and promote a great crust. This is an emmer khobz.

If the dough hasn't broken down too much, it can be slashed once to good effect.

Bake at 200°C for 30 minutes. The loaf will spread more than with wheat bread, form attractive rising cracks, and emerge brown and crusty.

For the tinned version, add a tablespoon more water when making the dough, so it is softer and also a bit more difficult to handle. Proof as for the crusty, but do the final rise in an oiled bread tin, which should be pre-warmed. Let it rise for at least 2 hours, until it is well risen and a bit critical and delicate with an extensively textured surface.

The loaf is much improved by sealing the tin with aluminium foil for the first twenty minutes of baking, then removing it to finish. A very "cakey" open crumb results which is soft and rustic.

Bake at 200°C for 30-35 minutes.

… I kept thinking of Rameses, Hatshepsut, Akhenaton any Pharaonic names I knew, shadowy figures who seemed closer and more real through eating the very same bread. And it makes melt in the mouth toast!

The Sourdough Loaf

EMMER FLATBREADS

To make Emmer flatbreads, using the recipe for emmer bread, divide the dough in two after the initial rise and roll each into a ball and leave to rest for a few minutes. Flour the surface well and gently, symmetrically, flatten the ball until it is a 1.5cm (½ inch) thick disk, "flatter" bread rather than "flat" like a pita bread. Turn it over as well so both sides are flat.

Place on an oiled or papered tray, brush with extra-virgin olive oil, extra-virgin sesame oil (best), a good nut oil or ghee. Leave to prove for 2 ½ hours, by which time they will be well fermented. Gently dimple them with your fingers and bake at 200°C for 15 minutes. Alternatively, griddle cook, even in a suitable barbecue.

Aromatics such as cumin seed, ajwain seed, coriander seed and fennel seed are often used to flavour these breads to good effect. Crush them slightly under a rolling pin to release their volatile flavour components before adding. 1-2 teaspoons per loaf is enough. Some people strew coarse rock salt on top before baking which gives a primordial tang.

Another savoury effect is to smear the flatbread with onion juice, and then salt immediately prior to baking. Grate an onion and squeeze through a sieve into a bowl to obtain the juice.

Rolled thinner still, these are obviously benchmark pizza bases, often still made in rural Italy where emmer has never gone out of fashion.

"Bread of the rings" (p 147) particularly applies to Emmer.

Following the Bread of the Rings method (pp 147 - 148), make a thick batter with emmer flour and water. Stir in 2 tablespoons of seed leaven, or start from scratch. It will be rampant in the morning or after about 8 hours.

Add sea salt and stir it in gently to ensure a uniform texture, leave 5 minutes to relax then spoon into the rings and griddle as described in the Bread of the Rings recipe. This makes really tasty unique and soft textured little breads - with lineage.

By adding very little bicarb soda, half a teaspoon along with the salt, the batter will thin a little and aerate more, making a pleasing cakey texture.

TROPICAL FRUIT BREAD

Ingredients.
- 400 g white bread flour.
- 200 g leaven, brown or white.
- 300 g tropical fruit juice.
- 50 g chopped dried banana.
- 50 g of one of: dried papaya, mango or pineapple, or a medley.
- 50 g dried dates, chopped.
- 5 g green cardamom pods.
- 3 g whole black pepper corns.
- 5 g cinnamon stick.
- 1 tbsp finely grated ginger root, or 1 heaped tsp of dried ginger powder.
- 5 g salt.

Glaze:
- Date syrup, carob molasses or honey.

This is an exotic bread, perfect smeared with home-made ghee or other luscious Indian dairy products such as rabri or malai, but equally good with quark, marscapone, clotted cream or just cream....drizzled with heady tropical honey.

The dried fruits are briefly soaked in fruit juice. There are a few tropical fruit juices available, and some blends, so choose the best unsweetened ones. Guava in the juice mix gives a really interesting touch, and there are also juices such as pineapple and coconut milk that are to be recommended, particularly organic pineapple and coconut. So if you choose, mix 100ml of coconut milk into the juice quantity.

The most common dried tropical fruits available are mango, pineapple, papaya and banana. Banana is a must really, and it is a fight between the rest with good dried mango hard to beat. Dried tropical fruits full of sugar, preservatives and colouring are best avoided, so check the ingredients.

Choose two fruit or do a micro mix of them all. I use dried dates in this recipe, but fresh medjool dates also really set this off. If using, do not soak them with the other fruit and add last to avoid them being over-mashed in all the mixing.

Method

First, warm the juice and soak the chosen dried fruits in it for 20 mins.

Grind the whole spices until a powder.

Drain the soaking fruit and pour syrup into the leaven and whisk to mix.

Add the flour, spices and salt and mix well. Form into a dough and knead briefly until a coherent soft dough forms. Add the fruit and mix in evenly.

Cover and keep warm, proof for 2 hours.

Then knead briefly by folding the dough a few times and shape into an oblong or round depending on basket type or tin. Place in a pre-warmed oiled tin or roll in flour and place in the basket/banneton/brotform.

Proof for 2 hours, a little more if necessary, it needs to be well-risen.

Bake at 200°C for the tin loaf for 35-40 minutes, and 25 minutes for a crusty loaf.

While still hot from the oven, brush liberally with the glaze.

This bread may also be risen in small cups and steamed in the way of puddings.

 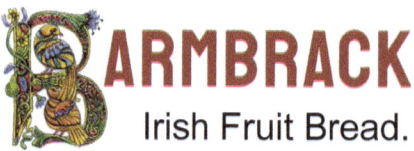 

Barmbrack
Irish Fruit Bread.

Ingredients.

- 400 g white bread flour.
- 200 g leaven.

The combination of white flour for the dough and sifted wholemeal (brown) for the leaven is most suitable.

- 50 g currants.
- 50 g sultanas.
- 50 g raisins.
- 2 heaped tsp tea in 300 g boiling water.
- 5 g caraway seed.
- 5 g sea salt.
- A thimble of best Irish whiskey (Optional).

Glaze:

- 1 tbsp liquid malt extract dissolved in 2 tbsp hot water.

My grandmother made a cake flavoured this way, spiked with caraway and the fruit soaked in tea. An Irish friend advised me to put in a cap full of best Irish whiskey while the fruit was soaking, and the bread seemed to rise an extra inch and had a special flavour. This is a very traditional version of barmbrack, even in Eire I couldn't find one which wasn't sugary and full of horrid peel, lacking in the delicious complexity of the fruit-driven fermentation.

Originally made with "barm", yeast scooped from brewing ale, this bread has great antiquity. Barm baking is a peculiarly Celtic-Gaulish practice which even astonished the bread-wise Romans when they conquered Gaul. The caraway flavouring has similarly ancient roots, being the oldest culinary spice identified, this from archaeological digs on Celtic settlements in Switzerland.

Associated with the ancient practice of Irish Halloween, barmbrack has an exciting character, almost unknown in breads. The Halloween brack traditionally contained various objects baked into the bread, and was used as a sort of fortune-telling game.

In the barmbrack were: a pea, a stick, a piece of cloth, a small coin (originally a silver sixpence) and a ring. Each item, when received in a slice, was supposed to carry a meaning to the person concerned: the pea, the person would not marry that year; the stick, the person would have an unhappy marriage or continually be in disputes; the cloth or rag, the person would

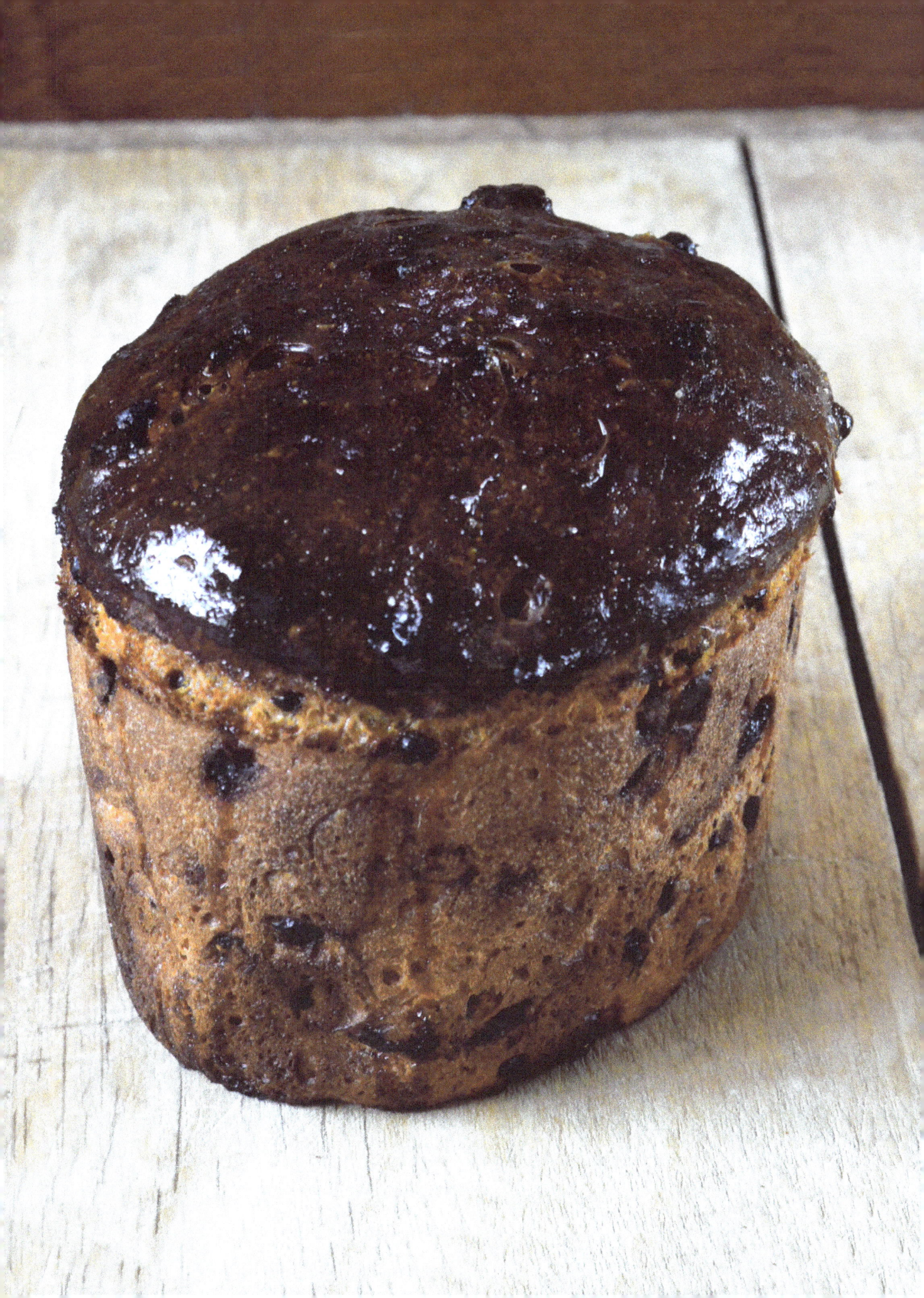

have bad luck or be poor; the coin, the person would enjoy good fortune or be rich; and the ring, the person would be wed within the year. Other articles added to the brack included a medallion, usually of the Virgin Mary to symbolise going into the priesthood or to the Nuns, although this tradition is not widely continued in the present day.

The barm process requiring brewing ale yeast is too complex to use here, and as I'm told by Irish critics that my brack is excellent, I'm guessing it was often made this way when the barm wasn't ready or available. This is the best of fruit breads.

I am reliably informed that brack was usually eaten with soft-ripened sheep or goat cheese (which are exceptional in Eire) and good ale, this being toothsomely brilliant. Slabs of sweet butter aren't far behind.

This recipe makes a loaf of 1 kg approximately, which can be a big crusty bread oozing tradition and unique aroma, with a worthy crust bursting with swollen charred fruit, or 2 smaller crusty or tin breads.

The quality of the dried fruit is significant, and if you intend to make this special bread, spend some time sourcing good dried fruit. When I first made barmbrack in Australia, it was possible to source beautiful plump purple currants which swelled in the soaking and bled imperial purple into the dough. This really referenced the gaelic meaning of "brack" which I'm told refers to the fruit as like a sparkling jewel in the crown of the bread - but why let the truth get in the way?

The magnificent purple currants have disappeared, as have the seeded muscatels which tasted of tempranillo, and I was never fully happy with the bread again. This was worse in the UK where the common (EU) currants are pin-sized which merely mocked the fruitiness and vanished into the dough, looking more like foreign bodies than glistening jewels.

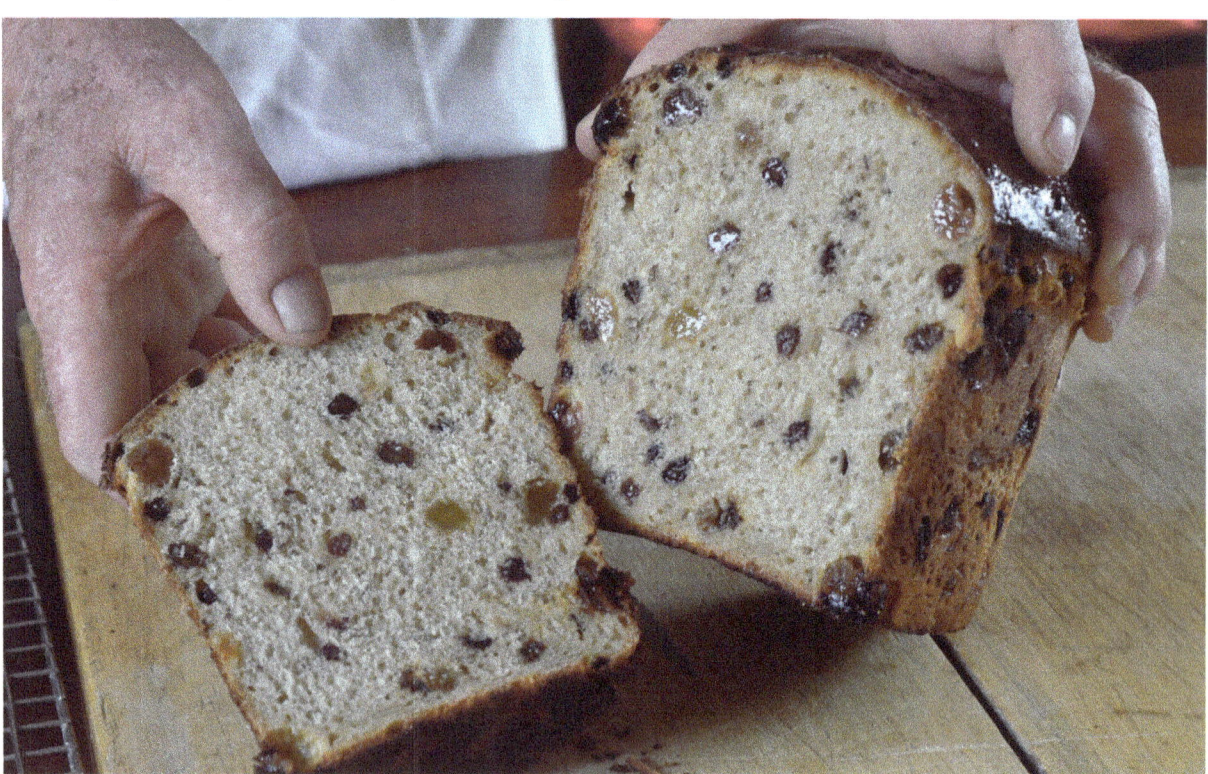

The Sourdough Loaf

The best dried fruit are called "natural or naturally dried", which means they are air dried, not sulphur-dried which leaches the colour of the fruit. Search for good fruit to make your efforts worthwhile and make this bread a real triumph. If really good fruit is not available, the bread can also be made with just one of the fruits. Treble the quantity, with good currants being ideal.

Tea bags will not produce the flavours in this recipe. By far the best is to brew tea from leaves, straining it into the fruit. The choice of tea is also important, choose your weapon, as smoky Darjeeling or Assam are like flavour-enzymes unleashing depth and character. Ordinary leaf tea also works well.

Brack can be made with white or sifted (brown) flour, the white flour version having greater volume.

Method

Start by making a nice cup of tea, which should be allowed to brew (my mother said "draw") for five minutes. Make sure to keep it hot. Strain it onto the dried fruit, add the whiskey if using it, and mix well. Cover and keep warm. Stir it every 10 minutes with a total soaking time 30 minutes or a bit more.

Strain the juice from the now fruity tea into the leaven and whisk until a bit frothy.

Add the flour, caraway and salt. Mix well until a smooth dough is formed, then fold the fruit through so it is evenly distributed. Cover and keep warm for 2 hours initial proof, by which time it should be well-risen and a bit sticky.

Re-knead it, gently folding it a few times, cover and rest for 5 minutes. Form into a round for crusty bread or an oblong for the tin. A spring-form cake-tin works well, in which case, form into a round and gently flatten to the edges. Cover, keep warm and leave to rise for a further 2 - 2½ hours by which time it will be rampant and ready to bake.

If necessary wait a further ½ hour as this needs to be well-risen. The tin needs to be baked at 200°C for 40 minutes, the crusty for 25 minutes.

As soon as it is out of the oven, on the wire rack and still hot, brush with plenty of malt glaze which will dry immediately leaving a shiny, oh-so-tasty crust.

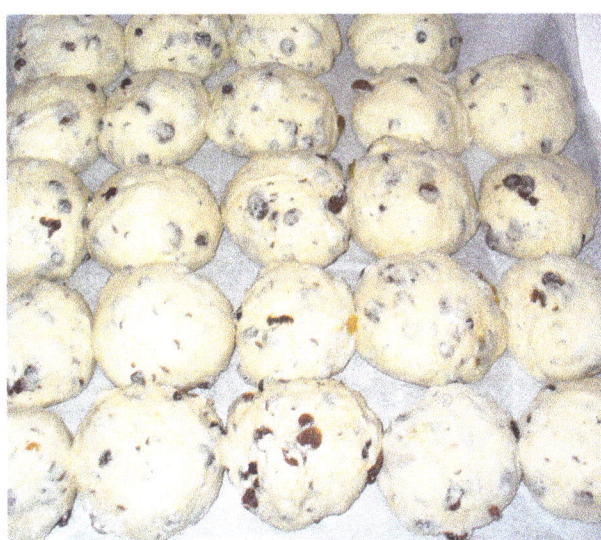
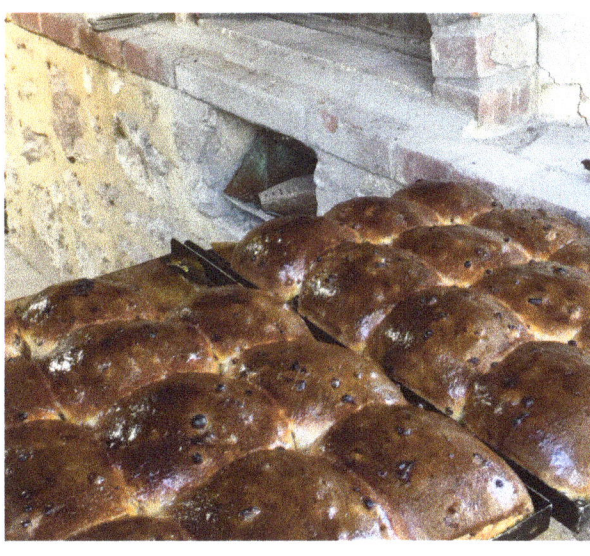

KURI AZUKI PAN

Chestnut and Azuki Bean Bread.

Ingredients.

Chestnut leaven:
- 145 g chestnut flour.
- 230 g water.
- 2 tbsp of stock leaven.

The bread:
- 500 g white bread flour.
- 375 g chestnut leaven.
- 180 g cooked azuki beans.
- 100 g azuki bean juice.
- 20 g sea salt.
- 100 g warm water (27°).

Chestnuts have always been a favourite since under-the-desk feasts of wild chestnuts while the teacher droned on, hot and charcoal-grilled from a street vendor in Hong Kong, exploding in the home oven, and the celebratory autumn dishes of Japanese cuisine I first encountered from macrobiotic teachers.

Chestnuts have lineage as important food from Europe to the Americas, being a staple for mountain folk in Europe for centuries. Most commonly used in castagnacchio, a rosemary and raisin infused dish from Tuscany; a bit-too-saccharine glacé marron from France; or even as a rare remnant of what was once English cooking as parsnip and chestnut "fritters", chestnuts were also incorporated into bread.

This bread is a mix of my influences really, and I was delighted to discover that chestnut flour ferments as a sourdough extremely well. It overcomes its slightly cloying nature, and in fact brings out the essential "chestnuttiness". It seemed natural to combine the chestnuts with azuki beans as is done in Japan - perfect partners.

Azuki beans are traditionally fortifying to the kidneys and when I first encountered them many years ago, they were called "sexy red beans" as in Traditional Chinese Medicine the kidneys (which they benefitted) are regarded as the source of libido.

As with food today, traditional combinations from different cultures are sometimes sublime, and this bread with a triple cream brie is a tour de force ... as it is with grilled tofu or roast duck.

The flavours evoked are novel, a mysterious synergy of mild cacao, spicey-savoury and sweet, fruity, of course nutty, with the azuki, a sanguine blush and the richly coloured dough as though speckled with raspberry. The dark crust is hugely appealing in flavour and texture, a perfect balance to the moist earthy crumb.

Method

Make a batter with chestnut flour and water, adding a little of the stock leaven. The flour absorbs a lot of water and on first peek the risen leaven reveals a much-fissured dome, almost exploding. Stir it down and leave to recover for a few hours.

Soak the azuki overnight, 8 hours, and bring to a boil, simmer until the beans are just soft, then add a pinch of salt. Strain and reserve the juice, drink whatever is left after making the bread, your kidneys will love you.

Mix the leaven with water and azuki juice, whisk to mix well, add the salt and flour. Mix well and knead for a few minutes until the dough comes together and is soft-springy, add the azuki beans and continue to knead until they are well incorporated.

Cover and prove for 2 hours, keeping it warm.

Turn out and re-knead briefly, form into a round, cover and let rest for a few minutes.

This is a ideally a crusty bread, so either re-round, roll in chestnut flour and place in basket, or flatten the round and roll into a tube to fit an oblong banneton/basket.

Pre-heat oven to 250°C. The final proof is for 3 hours by which stage it is well-risen. Turn out onto a hot baking sheet, shallowslash very gently, or leave to burst naturally.

As soon as the loaf goes in the oven, turn heat down to 200°C and bake for 20-25 minutes.

The bread fills the air with a wonderful spicy raisin-like aroma as it comes out of the oven.

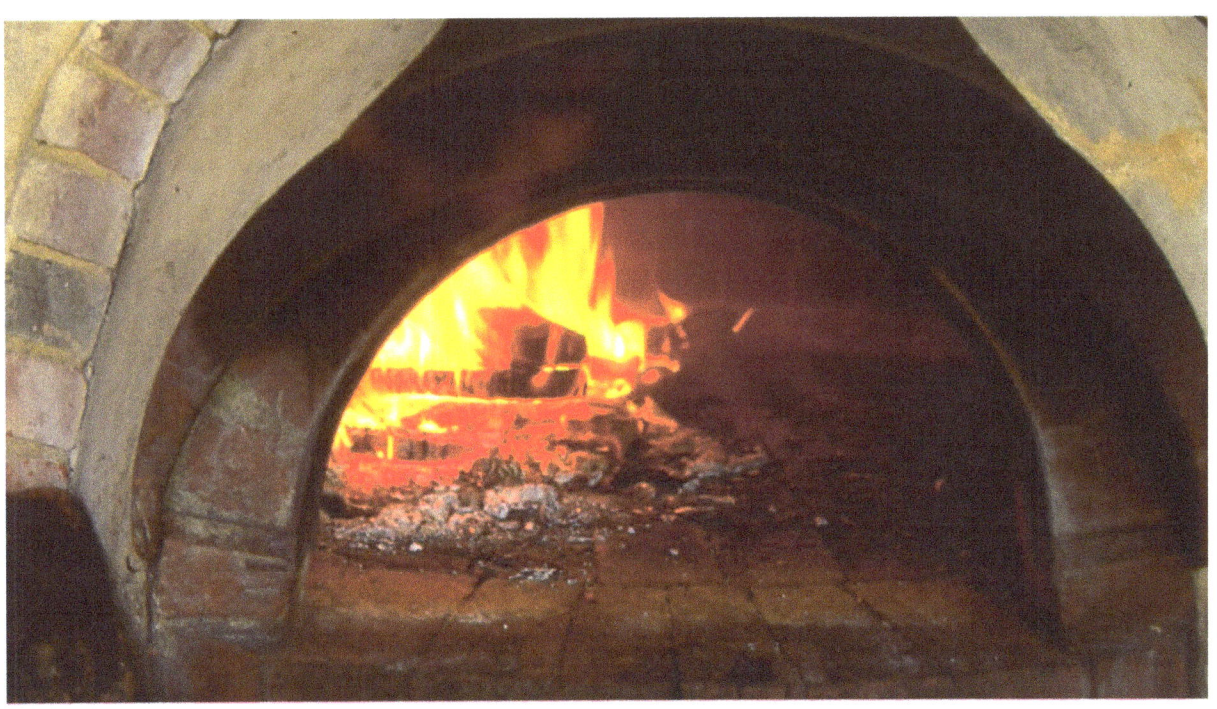

APPLE CIDER BREAD

Ingredients.

The leaven:
- 260 g wholemeal flour.
- 380 g freshly pressed apple juice, fermented.

The bread:
- 360 g wholemeal or sifted or white flour.
- 10 g sea salt.

The first "sourdough" I ever made, straight from the muse. Mildly flavoured, really simple, inherently organic, a true rustic bread.

It is made by pressing or juicing apples and allowing the juice to ferment. When the ferment is active, the flour is added to form a thick batter. This activates strongly and is the "leaven" and is used to make a dough. I simply couldn't believe this when it manifested all those years ago, and have wondered since, how many times this had been done in the past. It is clearly an alternative method of naturally fermenting a bread and developing a leaven.

On keeping this fruit ferment, and refreshing it with flour and water, it slowly morphs into an actual sourdough in that the bacterial component develops and all trace of the fruity-sweet yeasts disappear or are balanced by the development of the bacterial biome.

I had been cheffing, cooking really, in my busy groovy early 70s café, Byron Bay in the before time. The freshly pressed apple juice didn't get drunk... it was too busy, someone had driven from Sydney just to get my black bean mud crab, how could I turn him away?

The following day during lunch service, there was the apple juice with a foaming brownish head and full of sparkling bubbles. The muse allows no escape, there was a bag of freshly ground flour nearby, and then there was a leaven and then a dough, which rose quite rapidly in the warm humid air. It was in the oven, then emerging radiant on to a cooling rack in a blur. We all stared at this glowing russet loaf in disbelief and with a good deal of reverence. Could it really be that easy?

Method

To get the best results, use organic apples as there is more flora on the skins. Semi-tart or tart apples are best as very sweet ones easily go to an acetone ferment. Cider apples are perfect if available.

Depending on the ambient conditions, the juice will ferment overnight, but may take up to 3 days to really get going. This is a variable, wild yeast on bread street. Ensure to make extra juice for a taste, as it is so good when still sparkling.

As soon as the juice shows signs of fermentation - sparkles of bubbles, and a head - add the flour to form a thick batter. This will activate quickly if kept warm and will smell sweetly of yeast.

Add the flour and salt, mix well and knead to form a medium-soft dough, which will be more like a yeast dough than an edgy-sticky sourdough. This is because the ferment is largely yeast, just captured from the fruit, and the dough does not break down as a sourdough, because the bacterial component is missing. This also accounts for the relative sweetness of this bread, and for its lovely russet bloom.

Cover and keep warm until it is clearly fermenting and active. Usually 8 hours.

Add the flour and the sea salt. If using white flour, add a splash extra of juice.

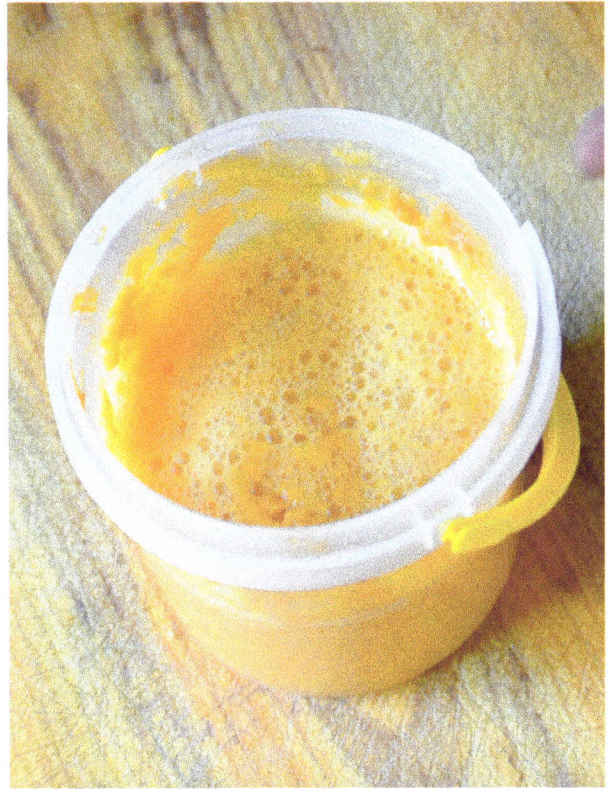

Mix the lot together to form a soft dough and knead for 2 minutes until clear with no unmixed lumps. Cover, keep warm and proof for 2 hours. Watch it as it may be ready after 1 hour if the right microbes are in residence. It should rise well and almost double in bulk. Gently reshape by folding, and form a round. Cover and rest 5 minutes. Re-round it and shape into either a round or oblong depending on how it will be baked, as a crusty or in a tin.

The next stage is usually 2 hours but keep watch. When well-risen, bake the tin at 200°C for 35 minutes. The crusty loaf will take 25 minutes at 200°C.

Add 2 tablespoons of freshly ground cinnamon for a cinnamon-toast bread, which is especially good as this bread has a close or cakey texture, being largely yeasty rather than the more developed or ripe texture of a sourdough. The residual hints of apple meld perfectly with cinnamon, especially when toasted. The cinnamon will slow the rise by about ½ hour.

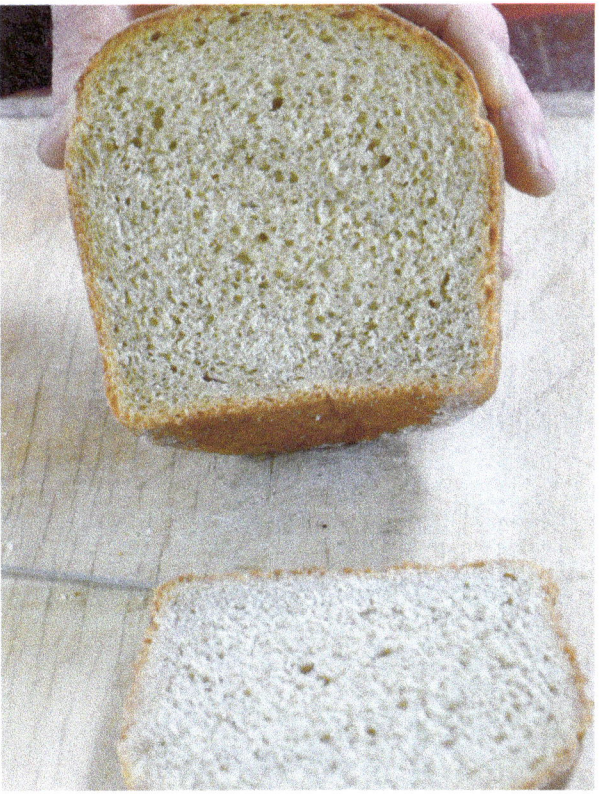

The Sourdough Loaf

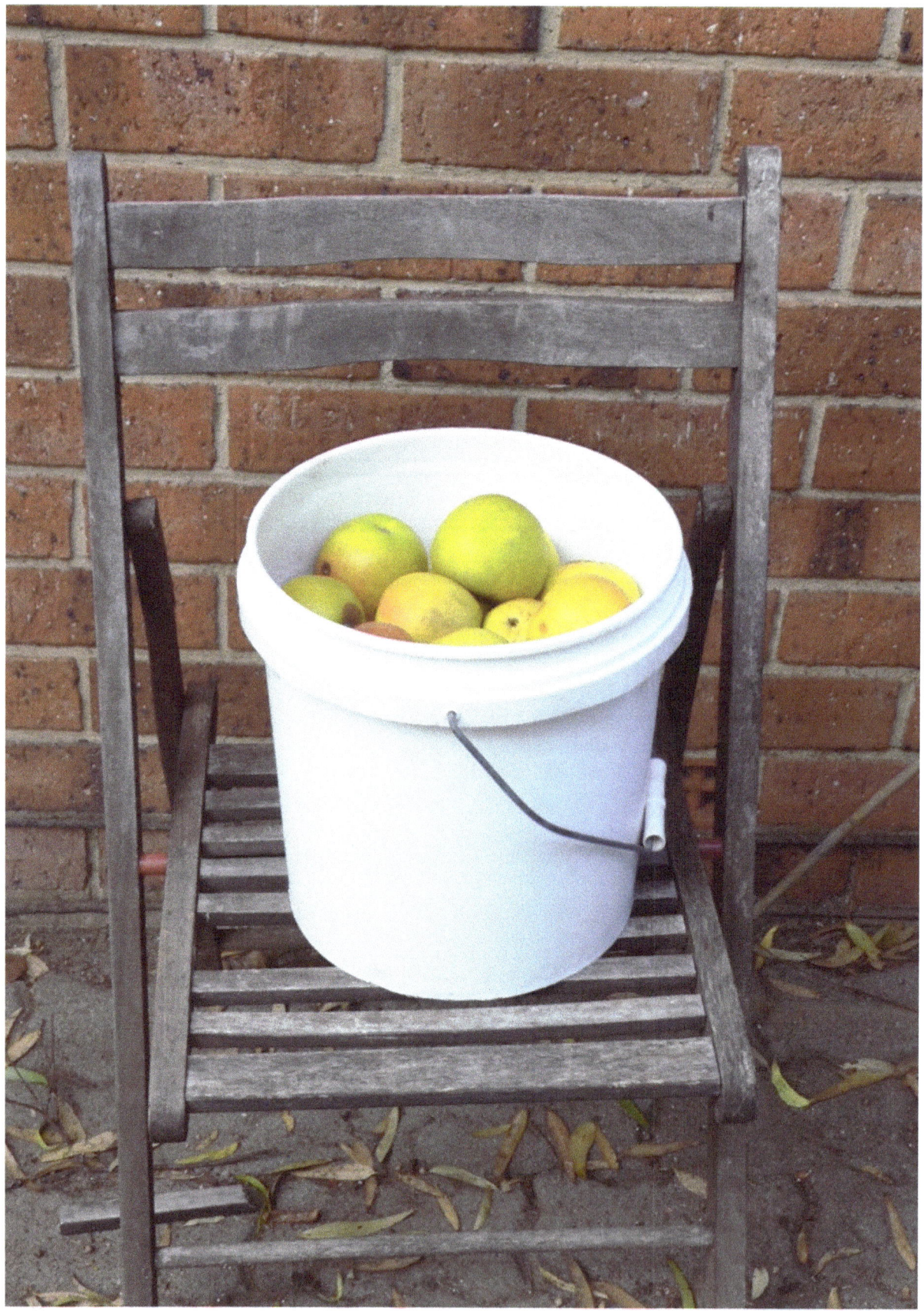

The Sourdough Loaf

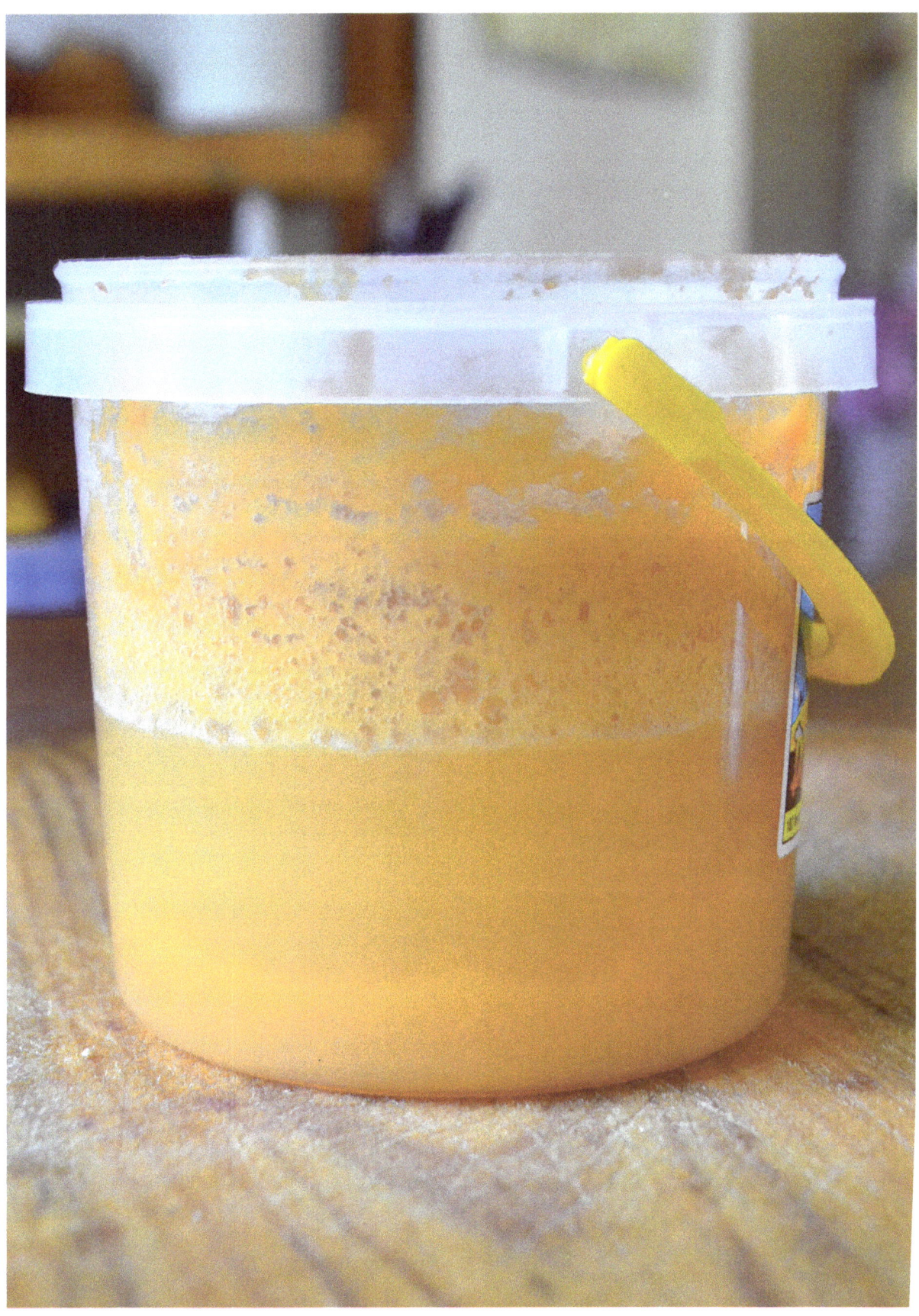

MUST BREAD

Ingredients.
- 2 kg of grapes.
- 400 g fermented grape juice.
- 600 g white bread flour.
- 5 g anise seeds.
- 5 g sea salt.

In the same way as the apple cider bread, this is a simple combination of fermenting grape juice and flour, traditionally with a hint of tiny anise seeds (not star anise). I am assured it is still made by some Grandmothers in the south of France, often as rusk for children.

The crumb-colour is pastel purple or lavender depending on the grapes, and the flavour is as surprising…distinctly of honey with the occasional aniseed spark…an unusual and ancient bread.

When grapes are crushed with the juice, prior to fermentation into wine, it is called must. If the skins and juice are dried, the yeasts which live on the grape-skins slumber and can be re-awakened to use as a leavening for bread. The Romans evidently used this method to preserve yeast, and it is still used today when dried raisins are soaked with flour to initiate a fermentation.

The grapes need to be organic or minimally spayed and as fresh as possible. Purple grapes such as Shiraz are ideal. The white bloom of yeasts is clearly visible on purple grapes.

Method
Crush the grapes and squeeze or press together with the skins, do not strain. Cover and leave to ferment somewhere cosy. In season, next to the vineyard, they burst into action overnight, breaking the surface formed by the broken skins with pink foam. This goes on for days, but peaks at about day 3, so the end of day 2 is a good time to use it for the bread.

Strain off the juice…drink some, it is the best sparkling wine I have tasted, and evidently in wine growing areas when wild fermentation was practiced, the whole hamlet would be woken or called as soon as the fermentation reached its heady peak. As with any sparkling alcohol, there was much merriment, as this brew carries the untamed Dionysian ether.

Mix all together and form into a smooth dough, which is easily kneadable. Knead for a few minutes, then cover it and keep warm. My surprise was that it ferments or inflates rapidly. Depending on how active the juice is, the dough usually doubles in bulk easily in 3 hours. Watch, and when it is double in volume, give it a thorough re-knead for a few minutes, shape into a ball, cover, keep warm and let rest for 5 minutes. This is a crusty bread, so shape into an oblong, or re-round it, roll in white flour and place in the basket. Cover, keep warm. This should be doubled in volume within the hour or perhaps 2.

Preheat the oven to 250°C.

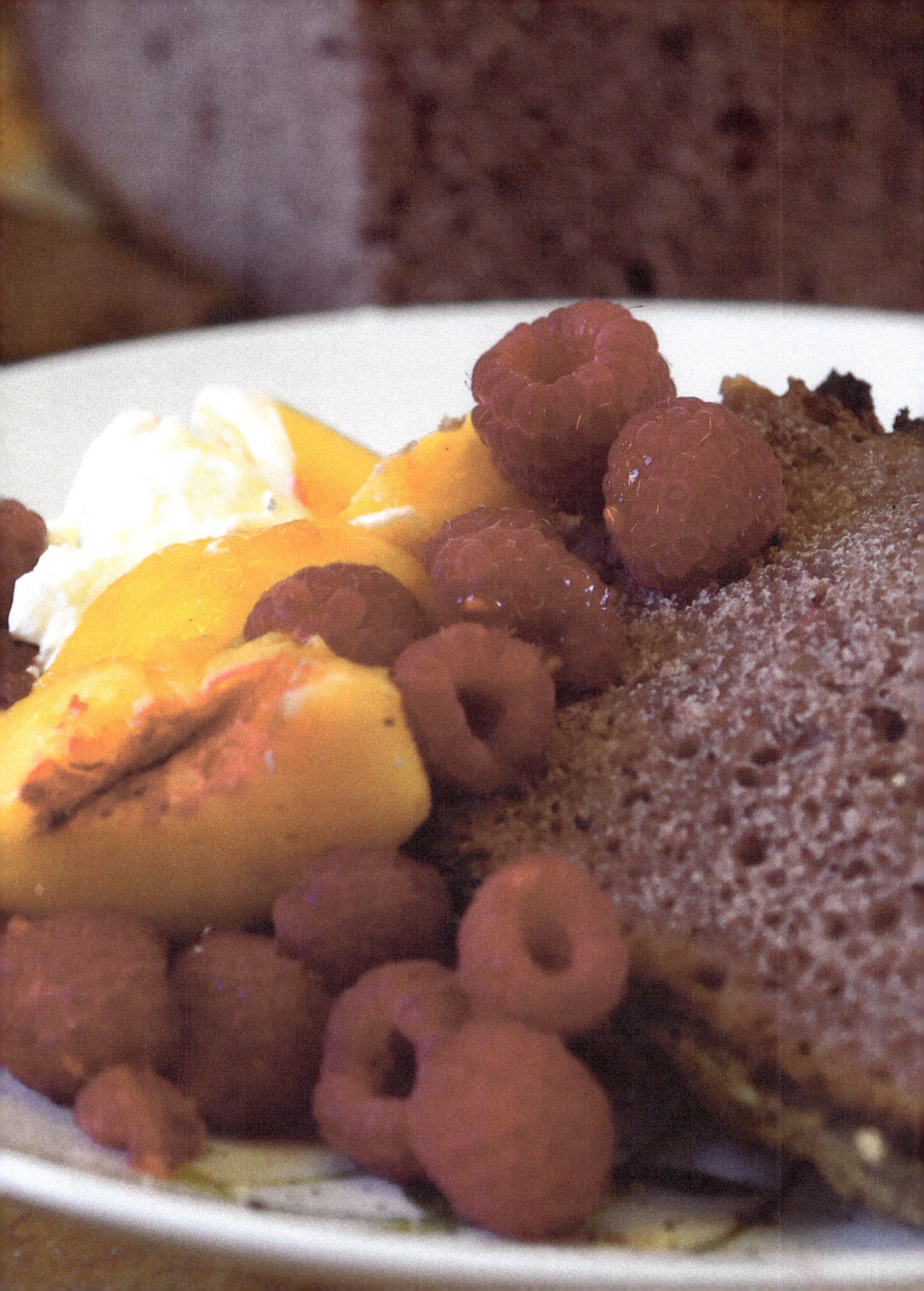

Slide the risen dough onto a hot tray, slash boldly. and reduce the heat to 200°C as soon as the loaf is in. Must bread usually has black to burnished tinges on its coloured crust and comes out of the oven with an overwhelming fruity air. Make sure it has a hollow ring when rapped firmly on the base, if in doubt bake for a few more minutes.

The texture is a little "woolly" and fragile when still warm, so tearing it is the best option at first. It is still brilliant the nest day.

I served must bread at a winery lunch with wild pine mushrooms grilled in the wood-fired oven, fresh goat's curd, and yellow peaches with a scarlet blush speckled with ruby-like pomegranate seeds.

If you cannot find real anise seeds, consider using a spoon of anise liquor, as the flavour is alchemic to this bread.

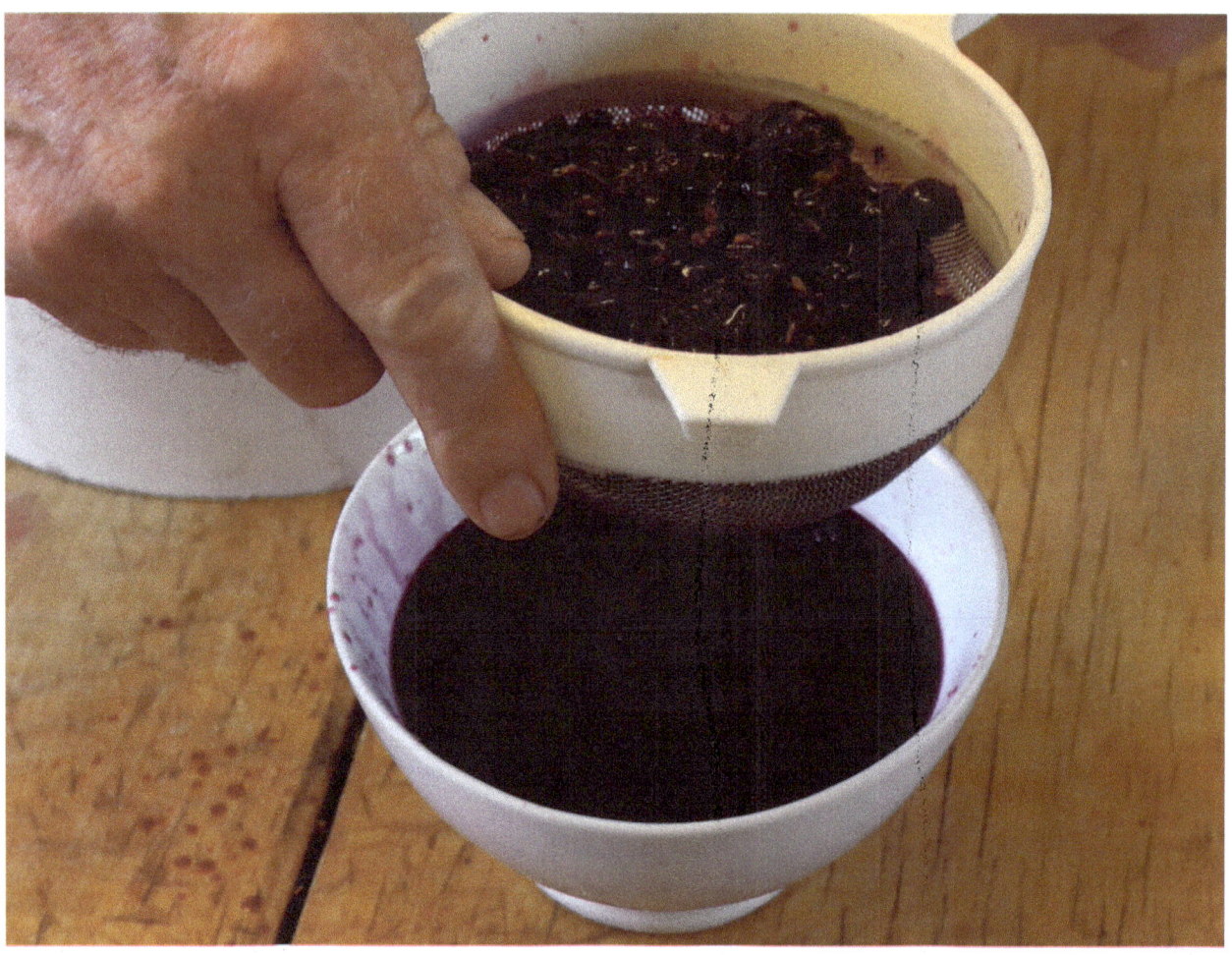

The Sourdough Loaf

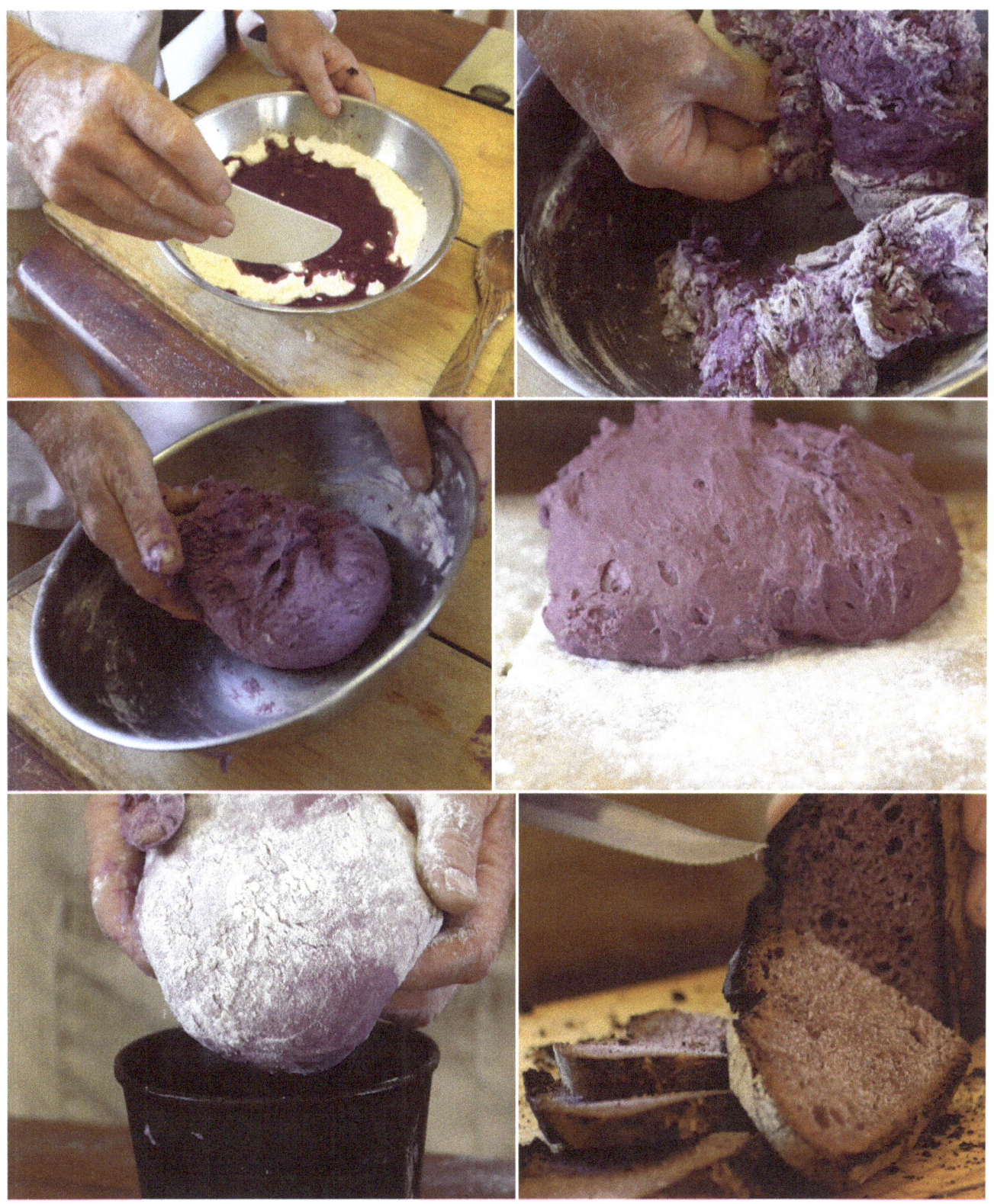

The Sourdough Loaf

PURPLE WHEAT AND YELLOW CORN BREAD

Ingredients.

- 280 g leaven.
- 300 g purple wheat flour.
- 125 g warm water.
- 7 g sea salt.

Sounds like the latest GM "super food" but purple wheat (formerly known as the artisan) has been around for a long time, so not intrinsically trendy, just new to us. It is a heritage wheat, as important as a heritage building. Evidently purple wheat evolved on the Ethiopian highlands, but red, yellow, white, blue, and black wheats were common in medieval Europe.

I purchased the purple wheat from a natural foods store.

Purple wheat is a part of the return to culinary reality, which represents variety, polyamoury of the plants, and a release from the relentless uniformity of agri-business controlled farming. Similarly, maize is multi-coloured, as are potatoes, tomatoes, and carrots and quinoa, and many many plants which have survived the singularity of the black hole of uniformity. When potatoes were white, flour was white, bread was white, and carrots were definitely all orange. They are now back to delight us, as the colour also represents a flavour.

When I first baked in the UK, it was surprising to make wholemeal, as the English wholemeal flour is generally very dark, the loaves looking more like rye. It was surprising because in Australia, wholemeal is yellow-golden, light brown, and clearly wholemeal yet nothing like UK wholemeal.

In the USA, some of the really strong wheat is very light in colour and produces quite a light-brown wholemeal. The US also has red wheat, the bran of which is colourful in a dough, and there is the famous English red lammas wheat, so different colours in wheat is actually common.

Undoubtedly purple wheat was used to make rustic sourdoughs and flatbreads, and this recipe will make an archaic "khobz" (cob), a round spreading loaf now common in North Africa, and usually made with white or yellow khorassan or durum flour.

Alternatively I have paired it with yellow corn meal, polenta, for amusement and to example variation in modern baking. Commercially, the punters love some variation, and this bread could be paired with virtually any other food to make a tempting and very delicious lunch. As with most good bread, it is exceptional with similarly rustic cheeses.

Purple wheat bread has a really attractive earthy flavour and it looks good as the purple holds in the finished loaf as a "purple shadow" tinged with tweedy flecks of yellow corn, if you are choosing to back the alternative note (instructions on the next page). The flavour is actually quite strong, almost mushroom-like and the bran is very tasty and unique.

Method

Make a purple wheat leaven in the same way as the original leaven instructions, using the purple wheat wholemeal and adding two tablespoons from your stock starter. This is very active in 8 hours, when it should be stirred. Wait for 3 hours for it to recover, at which time it should have risen up again and be clearly active.

Add the water to the leaven, whisk well, then add remaining ingredients. Mix well and knead for a few minutes until a pliable soft dough is formed. Cover, keep warm and proof for one hour.

Shape the dough into a high round, that is, it should not be flat as the loaf will spread. Roll in the purple flour and place on an oiled or papered baking sheet, with any seams or cracks on the bottom, leaving a domed surface to rise.

My practice is to invert a bowl over the loaf, big enough so that when the loaf spreads it will have plenty of room. In any case, cover, keep warm and allow to prove for 1 ½ hours by which time it will have spread and be showing some breaking bubbles and a few fissures . Bake at 200°C for 30 minutes.

This is a great "break and eat" bread, not with industrial superstructure, to be enjoyed with a thick soup or a tagine.

With yellow corn:

Pour 120 g of boiling water on to 80 g of coarse yellow corn meal and a good pinch of salt, while stirring to avoid lumps. Leave it to settle for 1 hour.

When the above purple wheat dough has had its initial proof for 1 hour, chop it into 6 or so pieces and mix well with the soaked corn meal and 50g of extra purple wheat flour, dusting the surface lightly with flour. Re-knead gently until a soft almost sticky dough is formed. Form into a round, cover and leave to recover for a few minutes.

This loaf is quite soft and may be risen in a tin or follow the khobz procedure. Roll the relaxed dough into a cylinder, roll in cornmeal and place in a warmed tin with any seams on the bottom. If making a crusty loaf, roll in coarse yellow corn meal.

Cover, keep warm and leave to rise for 2-2½ hours, by which time it should be quite delicate and well-risen.

Bake the crusty at 200°C for 30 minutes, a tin for 40 minutes.

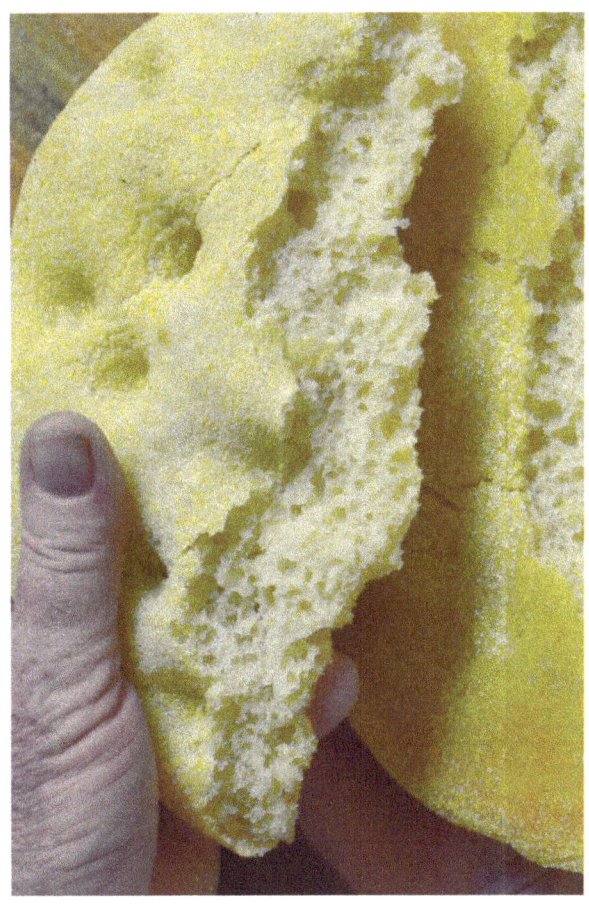

RICE BREAD
Gluten Free Bread.

Ingredients.

Leaven:
- 150 g brown rice flour.
- 50 g chickpea (besan) flour.
- 240 g water.
- 2 tbsp stock leaven.

The bread:
- 275 g white rice flour.
- 100 g chickpea flour.
- 420 g brown rice/besan leaven...this should be a very thick batter, not liquid at all.
- 300 g warm water (25°).
- 20 g sea salt.

(Makes 2 small loaves or 1 large)

This is a really palatable bread, and avoids the gums and artifice of most gluten-free breads. It is also more nutritionally balanced than some gluten-free concoctions and very digestible for that poor irritated tummy. While having a mildly strong flavour, but no more than a mild cheese, this bread has a soft moist texture not unlike good white bread! It will not win a competition for external panary perfection, but I like its rugged reddish- colourful crust.

Besides adding balance of protein to the rice, the chick pea (besan) flour contributes its own mellow and appealing flavour, tempered from any beany taint by the fermentation.

Method

The leaven, as always, is a key to the success here, and the leaven made from brown rice flour and besan is very active, as is the rise of the bread, surprisingly so.

The leaven is initiated with a little of stock leaven, which will be made from wheat flour. If this is a worry to those wanting to avoid any taint, a leaven can be initiated using brown rice and chick pea flour, simply follow the leaven making instructions (see pp 40 - 47), but substitute these two flours at the ratio of 3 times brown rice to besan. The leaven batter will need to be a little firmer however....or, re-make the seeded leaven a second time, just using the brown rice and besan, by which time any residual gluten will be well gone. Brown rice flour can vary, so if the batter seems thin, use more flour.

Ferment at least 8 hours or until clearly active and rising up in the container....best not to let the ferment drop, but catch it when most active.

Add the leaven to the water and whisk it, followed by the flours and salt.

This is not a kneading proposition, simply mix it well and give a thorough stir until stiff but creamy.

Scoop it with the slip into a pre-warmed, well-oiled tin, smooth the top with the slip. Cover and keep warm. It will be double in size after 2-2½ hours. Do not ferment further as it will collapse somewhat, with a sagged top crust….the bread will still be fine however.

Bake at 200°C for 35 minutes until it gives the nice hollow sound when rapped. Bake a further 10 minutes if you aren't satisfied.

An alternative to a tin loaf is to place the dough on a baking tray with 4 sides, and allow it to spread and ferment well; it is a good focaccia-style slab. While proving, brush the top with plenty of extra-virgin olive oil or extra-virgin sesame oil to maintain a soft and tasty crust.

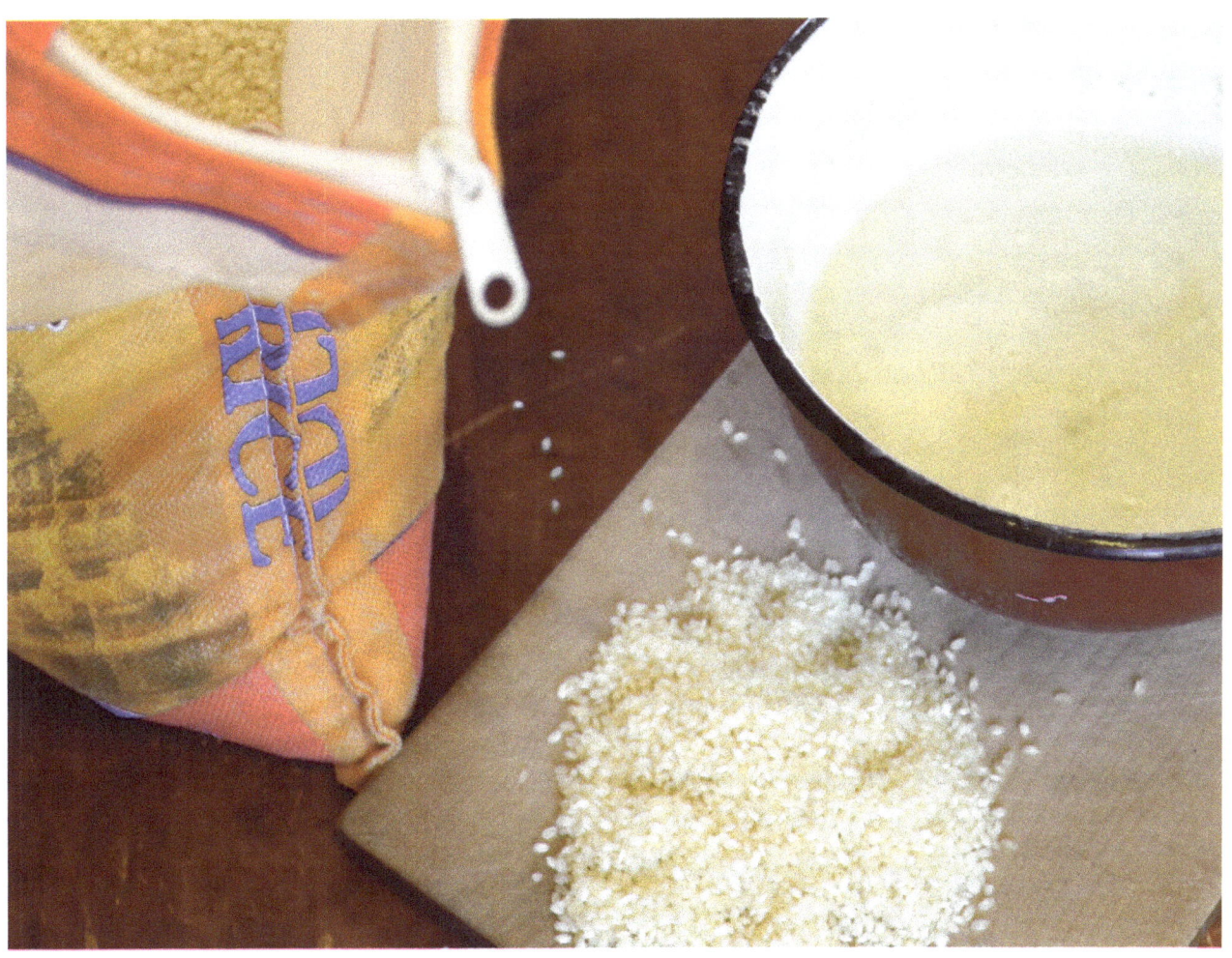

GINGER BREAD

Ingredients.

Spice mix:
- 3 tbsp ground ginger.
- 1 tbsp ground cinnamon.
- 1 tsp anise seeds.
- 1 tsp coriander seeds.
- 1 tsp cardamom pods.
- ½ tsp cloves
- 1 tsp allspice.
- ½ tsp ground nutmeg.
- 1 tsp fennel seeds.
- 3 tsp pepper corns.
- 1 tbsp licquorice powder.

The bread:
- 400 g sifted wholemeal flour.
- 100 g rye flour.
- 270 g warm water.
- 250 g leaven.
- 10g salt.

This is an ancient devotional bread evidently from Armenia, the original Christian nation. The mixture of nine spices commonly used in medieval times was thought to be *'the perfect praise of god', 'the holy trinity, the three elements and the three spheres'.* The ginger breads had many forms as biscuits or cake or bread, with the biscuits or crackers in the shape of a bishop (Saint Nicholas), or as 'icon' shapes, pressed from a beautifully carved wooden mould.

Recent recipes all contain baking powder or soda, which wasn't around until the 19th century, so I am sure ginger breads were originally sourdough. The breads also contained quite a bit of rye flour, depending on the harvest and locality.

Symbolism and imagery are indeed different today. Decorate them or form as you wish, anthromorphic or geometric. This version is risen in a baking tray, rolled or pressed out 5cm thick, and it will double in bulk to form a risen biscuit slab. Once it is rolled into the tray, slice deeply in the required shapes.

This spice mix has eleven spices, but use any of the spices combined to make 5 tablespoons. The basic most important spices are ginger, cinnamon and cardamom, with the licquorice powder giving a unique and authentic touch.

This makes quite a lot of ginger bread, but why not?...share it around. In any case, it keeps so well and matures perfectly - in 2 months time you will be glad!

Method

Follow the crusty bread method (pp 81 - 84) for baking instructions. Add the spices as a last step.

Grind all the seeds to a powder and mix with the pre-ground spices.

This will be slower to proof as the spices slow it all down. Keep it covered and warm for 2-3 hours.

Roll out or press out to 1.5cm thick with the rye flour and place in the well-oiled or papered baking tray, or two, and cut deeply into shapes or squares.

Alternatively, roll out and cut with shapes.

Cover and keep warm. It should double in bulk in two hours, or leave it overnight at ambient temperature.

Bake at 200°C for 20 minutes. Immediately when it is out of the oven and still hot, spread on 1 cup of best honey, set aside and leave to cure for 12 hours.

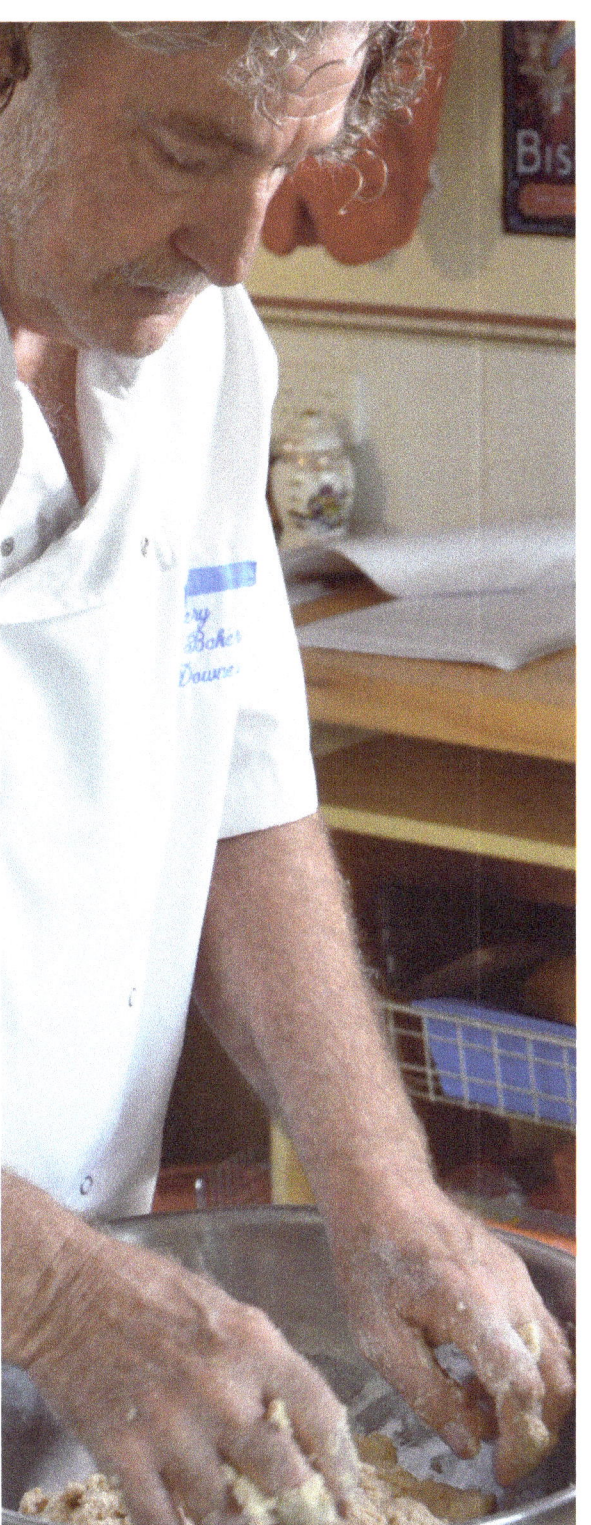

BARM BREAD

This is a 3 stage recipe, with ingredients added at each stage:

The night before:
- 250 g wholemeal flour.
- 200 g water.
- ½ tsp organic or dried yeast or 1 tsp compressed yeast.

The next day:
- 500 g wholemeal flour.
- 600 g water.
- 1 tsp salt.
- 1 tbsp malt extract.

Plus:
- 800 g wholemeal flour.
- 250 g (1 cup) warm water.
- 1 heaped tbsp salt.

Although not a sourdough, this bread has an ancient lineage and is well worth making because of its superb flavour and texture. Similar to sourdough it has a lengthy fermentation but without the "twang" or acidity of sourdough. It was the preferred bread of much of the British Isles.

It is so good and ancient, that Pliny mentions it in his work on Gaul, written after Julius Caesar's initial incursions into the Celtic world. The bread savvy Romans were astonished by this bread, leavened with ale-yeast.

The old practice popular in the British Isles until the 1950s was to scoop the top froth of yeast from brewing ale (not lager) and then either directly pitch it into the dough or to wash and store it for later use.

When working in the UK I discovered a way to make it for the home baker. This was enabled by the production of organic yeast in Germany. This yeast is not the line-bread diabetic yeast dependant on sugar, but a robust yeast which will grow with the vigour required.

It can be done with commercial dried yeast, but I have had this die on me half way through the process. It can also be made with commercial compressed yeast, but the German organic yeast is a clear winner. Using an ale yeast from a brewing store mixed with compressed yeast can also be successful.

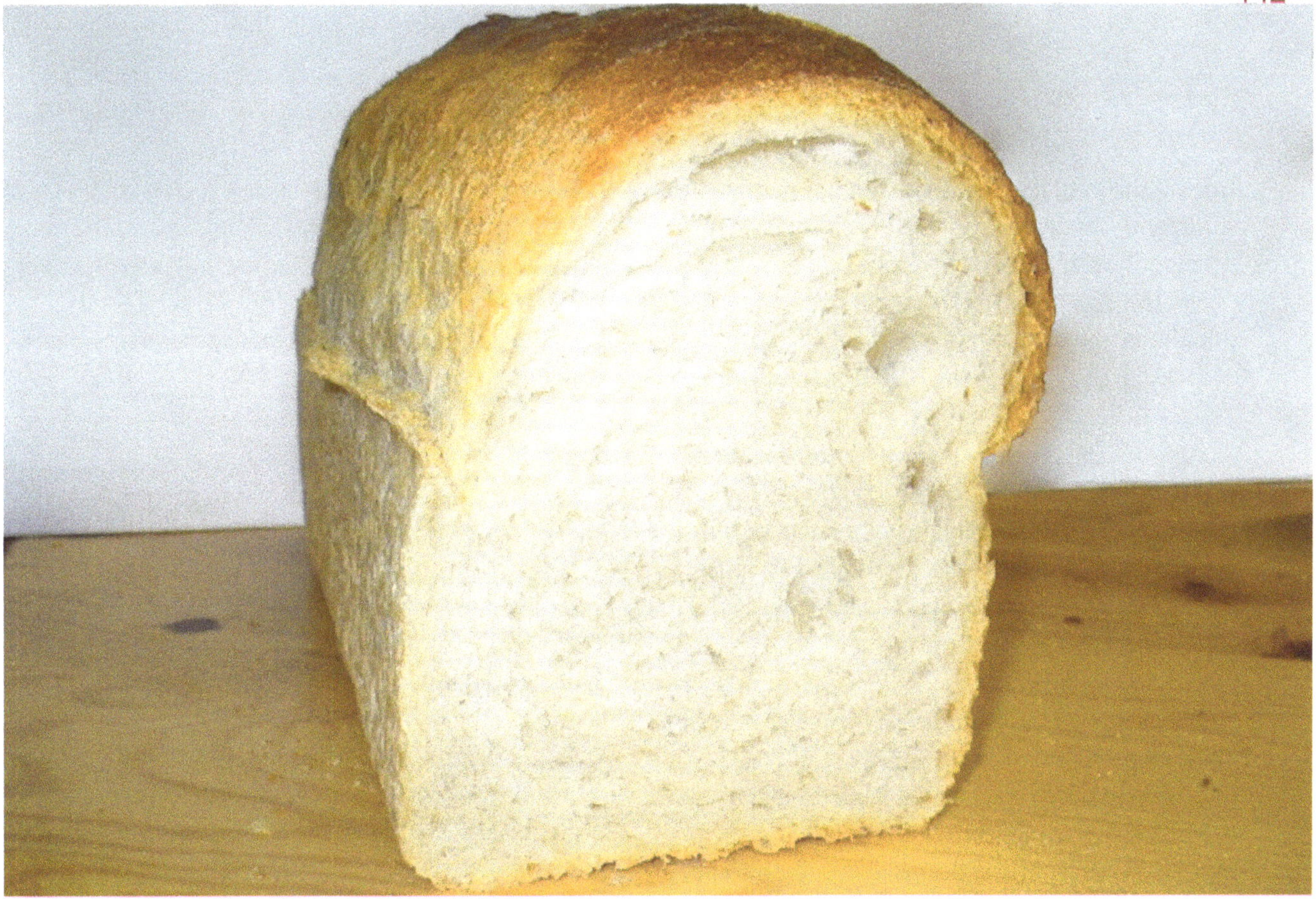

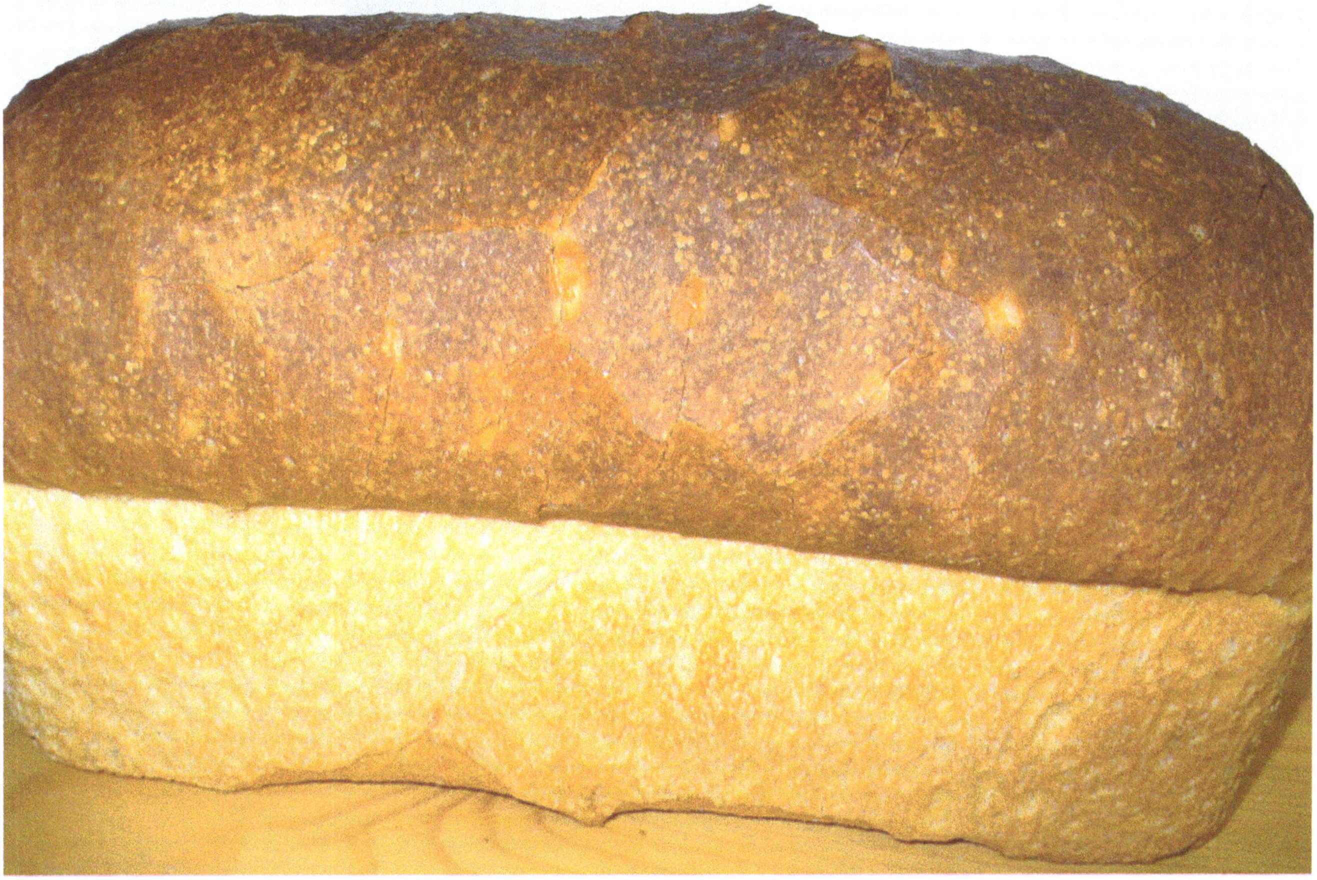

During the long fermentation, the flour is sufficiently hydrated and a mild acidity is developed which makes the bread very digestible, and being a sourdough baker myself, I felt almost guilty preferring this some days to my sourdough.

Sometimes the brewing yeast was unpredictable and just "went off", clearly the root of "barmy" when applied to a person! Barm bread makes superb toast, much commented on by European visitors in past times, and barm cakes were a regional specialty in the north of the UK.

I got this bread into commercial production in the UK and it was much commented upon. This encouraged me to make it available to home bakers, as it is well worth making. While it is more difficult than sourdough, it is truly part of the ancient craft of baking bread.

This process also enables the very best crust…EVER…and was the required method for the best cottage loaves, a famous English crusty bread, and today, it makes the best baguette…EVER as well.

This method employs what in British baking is called a sponge. It is not the same as a poolish, often and previously used in French and Viennese baking. The major difference here is that the yeast is directly pitched into a poolish batter.

The sponge is made from yeast which is previously grown in a firm dough, and this sponge, in the very ancient manner, contains barley malt which really distinguishes it and sets up the correct flavour profile, as the barm was originally raised in a wort made from barley malt.

Method

As mentioned, before yeast was industrialised, most English/Scottish/Irish bread was made with yeast scooped from the top of fermenting ale. This recipe replicates that process. If you can't source the organic yeast, use regular, preferably compressed, yeast and buy some ale-type yeast from a brewing store to pitch in with it. Otherwise just use dried yeast but the results won't be the same, flavour-wise. Use 1 teaspoon of the brew-store yeast mixed with the other yeast you employ.

This makes a large loaf, which I like and is traditional but make two smaller loaves if preferred. Next time you will double the recipe as it is so good, and keeps very well. Smaller loaves require less baking time.

The night before: Mix ingredients well into a firm dough ball. Cover with a plastic bag to prevent drying out. Place in a not-cold spot and leave overnight to activate.

The next day: When the dough is clearly active mix together with the wholemeal flour and warm water, salt and malt extract. (Mix the malt with the water for ease of process.) Mix until clear, cover, set aside in a warm spot for 4 hours or until a very active batter. This is the sponge.

Plus: Mix the sponge with wholemeal flour, warm water and salt. Knead/mix into a smooth dough, cover and set aside for 1 hour, by then it should be clearly rising.

Give it a good knead, rest for 5 minutes, then roll into a cylinder and place in a well-oiled warmed tin, in a warm spot (important) to rise. The top should be smooth with no cracks or fissures. This will take 45 minutes to one hour, by which time it should have reached the top of the tin. Bake at 250°C for 15 minutes, then 220°C for 45 minutes more.

There should be a good oven-spring, resulting in a well-risen bread with a high top.
Hopefully it all worked and the bread should have a very appetising aroma, with a nice dark upper-crust. It should be an archetype of good bread.

Alternatively, this bread can be made with unbleached white flour or a sifted wholemeal, which is the traditional "brown" bread. You will have to finesse the textures a bit, but it works.

It is best to use the softest flour available for the final flour addition. A cake flour works perfectly and helps to impart the finest flavour.

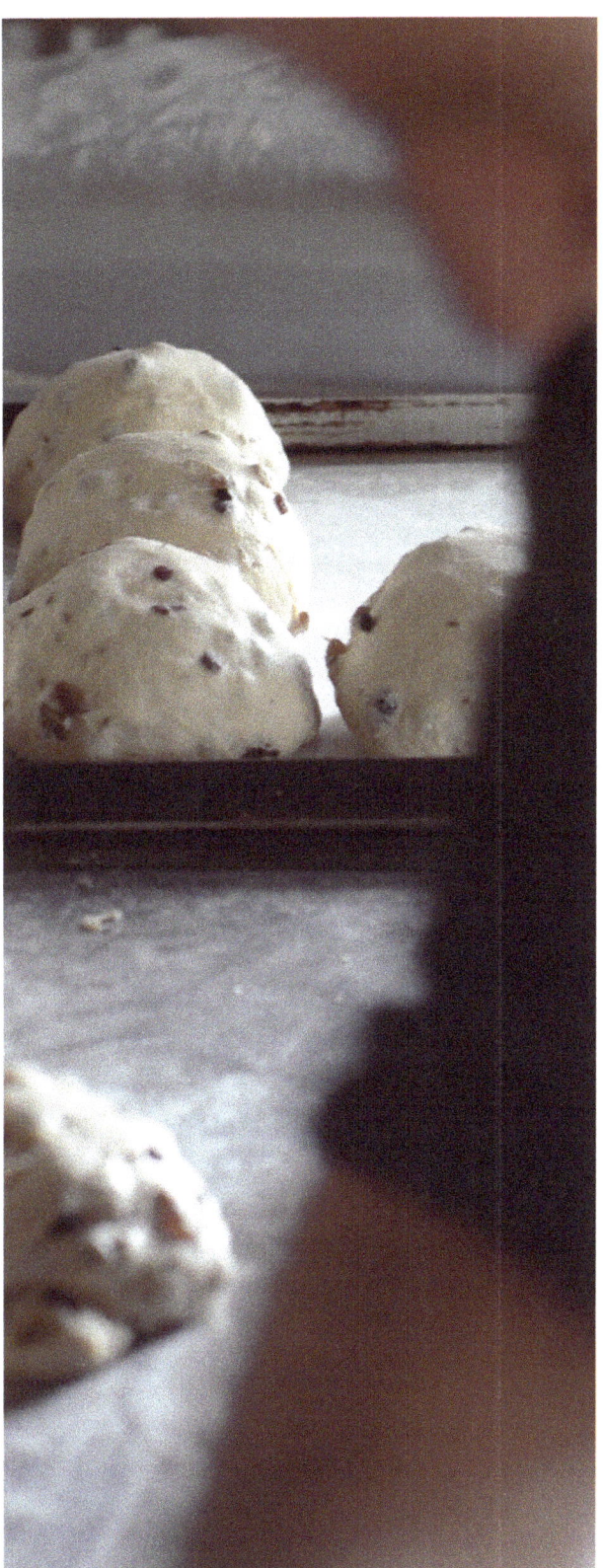

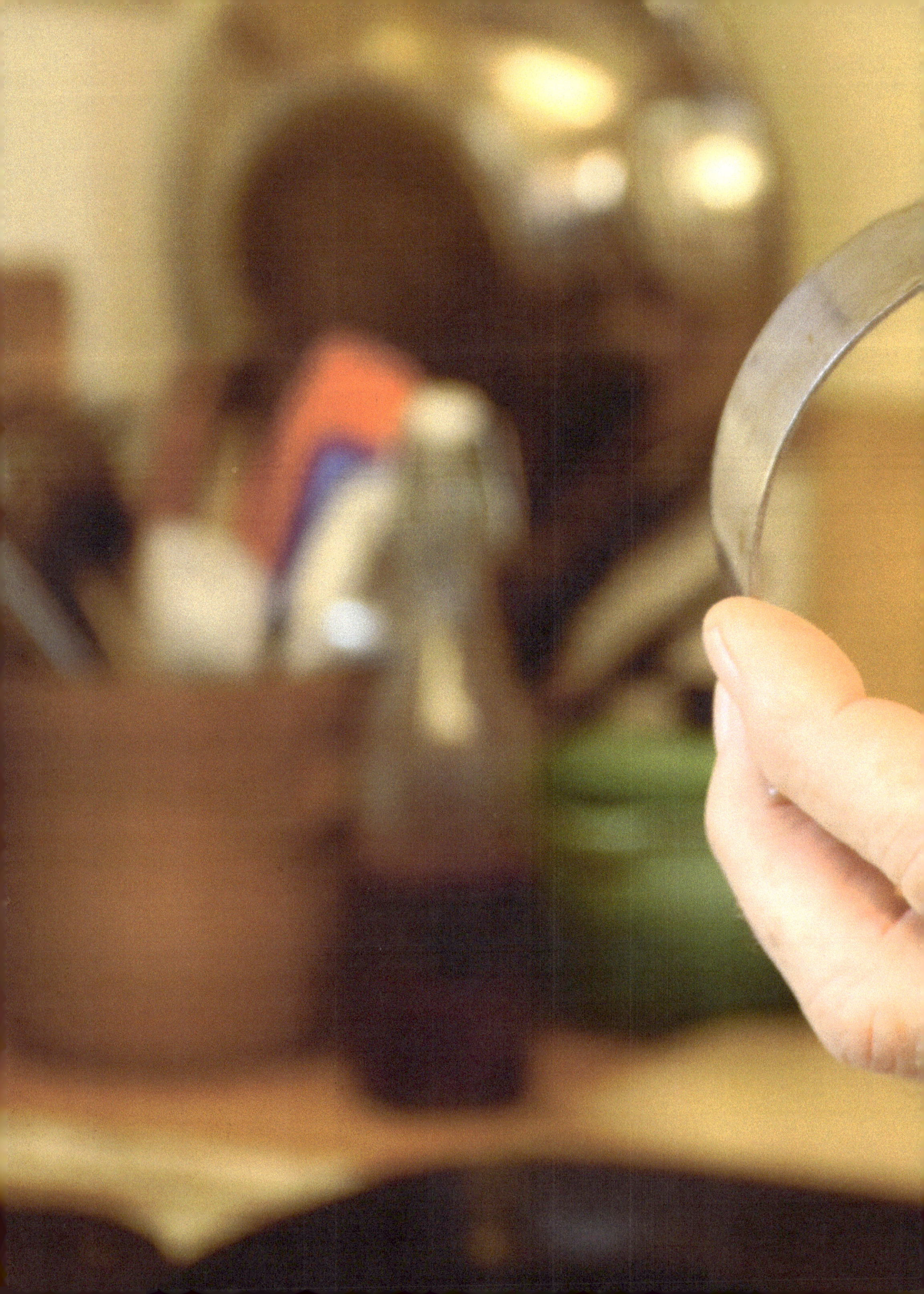

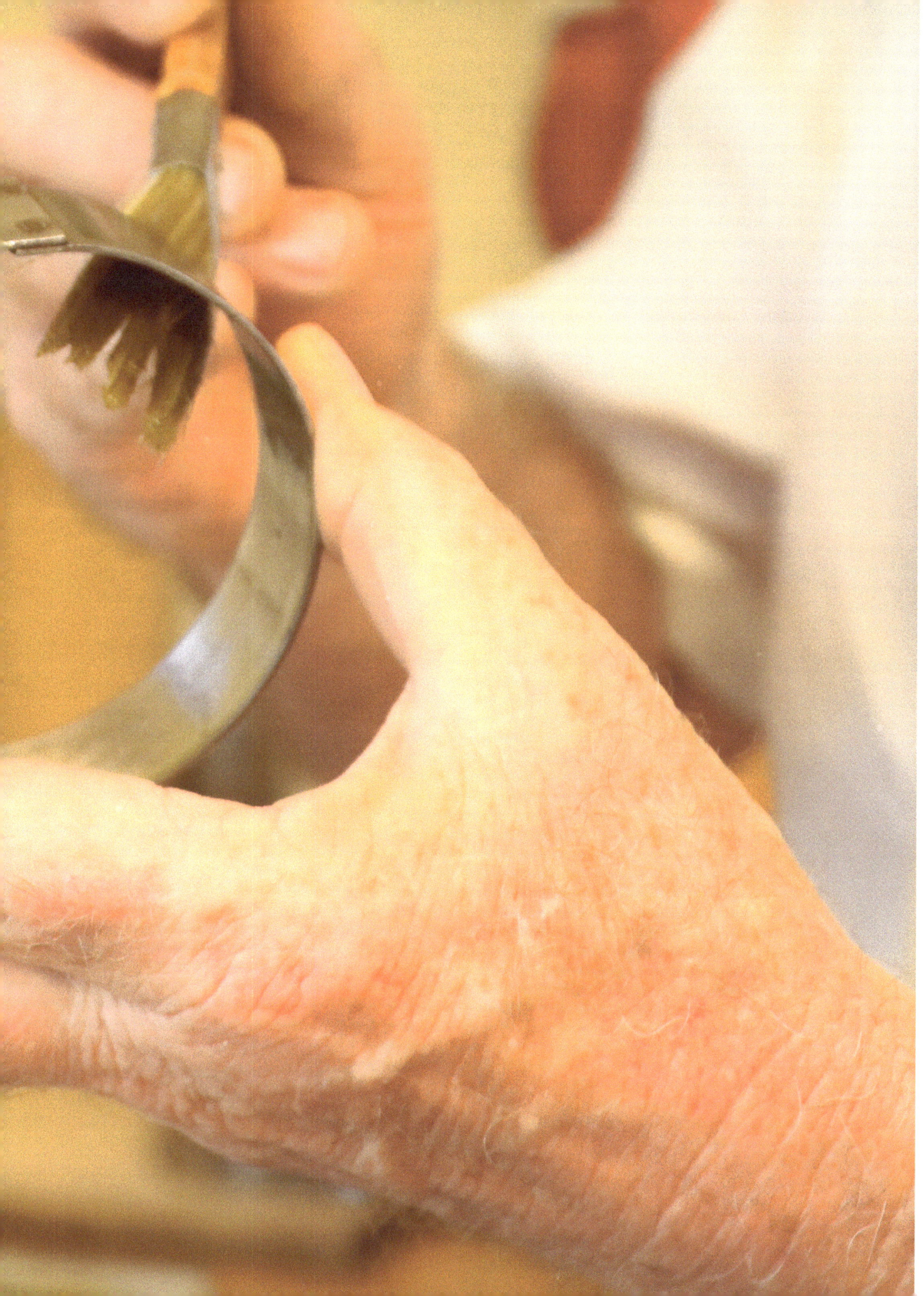

BREAD OF THE RINGS

In the before time, bread clearly started in the ashes, as can be seen from an existent ancient culture, this indigenous Australian Pitantjatjara woman from the central desert (APY lands), is making an incredibly nutritious (and tasty) bread from purslane seeds with an age-old technique.

The technique is to wet-grind the seeds to form a thick paste which is carefully deposited in the ashes, but not just any ashes, only certain wood burns to a suitable soft white ash atop glowing coals. Roman history describes focaccia being made in the same way, "focaccia" means *baked in the ashes*, or *hearth bread*. Keep it in mind for the next camping trip.

An alternative step in the evolution of bread, apart from the wood-fired oven and the cloche, was to make bread on a metal griddle or girdle with these batters. The griddle is usually made from iron, often round and was common from India (tava) to Eire (girdle). Cleaner than the ashes and less fuss or urban than an oven, these were the bread irons of people who were accustomed to move rather than build cities, an ancient cultural signifier.

The batters survive as enriched pancakes, crepes, pikelets and crumpets, but behind these surviving forms is a simple technique for easily making batter breads.

For example, the wholemeal leaven recipe if made thicker, but still a batter like the pitantjatjara bread, can be baked in the ashes or on a hot stone or griddle or pan. It must be leavened bread genesis.

The thick batter may also be confined within a metal ring or hoop on the griddle and attractive round breads can be made, crumpet-like from the common cereals of barley, oats and chickpeas, and others now less common such as buckwheat and millet.

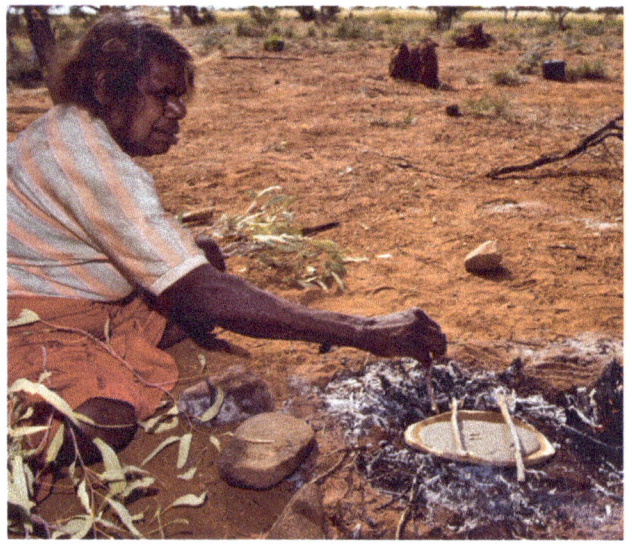

It always seemed hard to get a gastronomic fix on just how we ate so much barley (especially) and oats, for thousands of years. Easy to denigrate as gruel, and possibly that's true, but there were methods of making bread on griddles that were widely done, sometimes intensely locally, in England, Scotland and Eire, indeed everywhere.

Usually the fermenting is not recorded, or it is said the dough was rested or left to "turn", and the culinary history and practice largely lost.

Simply fermenting the batter and baking it directly on the griddle, as "cakes" was common. Indeed, barley cakes made in this way, and with the aid of a metal ring are exceptionally good, as are oat cakes and chickpea cakes, and those made with the ancient common grain, emmer wheat.

The Sourdough Loaf

A "modern" development which improves aeration and virtually eliminates overt sourness, is to add a tiny amount of bicarb soda to the batter before baking on the griddle.... clearly the original use of bicarb in baking, as the organic acids in the sourdough react with the alkaline bicarbonate producing gas.

This is an easy, low-skilled quick way to make good sourdough bread using very low and no-gluten ingredients. The barley and oat breads are delicious and sustaining, exceptional even with any good cheese, which is their culinary "evolutionary niche".

As rounds, quite a lot can be made with no fuss or bread-making-neuroses, and they perform the culinary function of a roll in a way, easily sliced through or stacked and filled with meats, cheeses, salads, or toasted with honey and butter, or as accompaniments to a serious wintery stew, or stacked and adorned post-modernly with amazing saucey vegetables, wild mushrooms and herbs.

Clearly, "bread" does not have to conform to the imprint of the white risen baked item.

One of my favourite authours and an erudite gastronome, Elizabeth David reports this telling local technique in "English bread and yeast cookery", arguably the best-ever book on bread: *"Yorkshire oatcakes. Originally the leavening was not ale-yeast but a spontaneous leaven made from an oatmeal sourdough..."*

The following recipes contain a selection of delicious sourdoughs that riff off this "Bread of the Rings" theme.

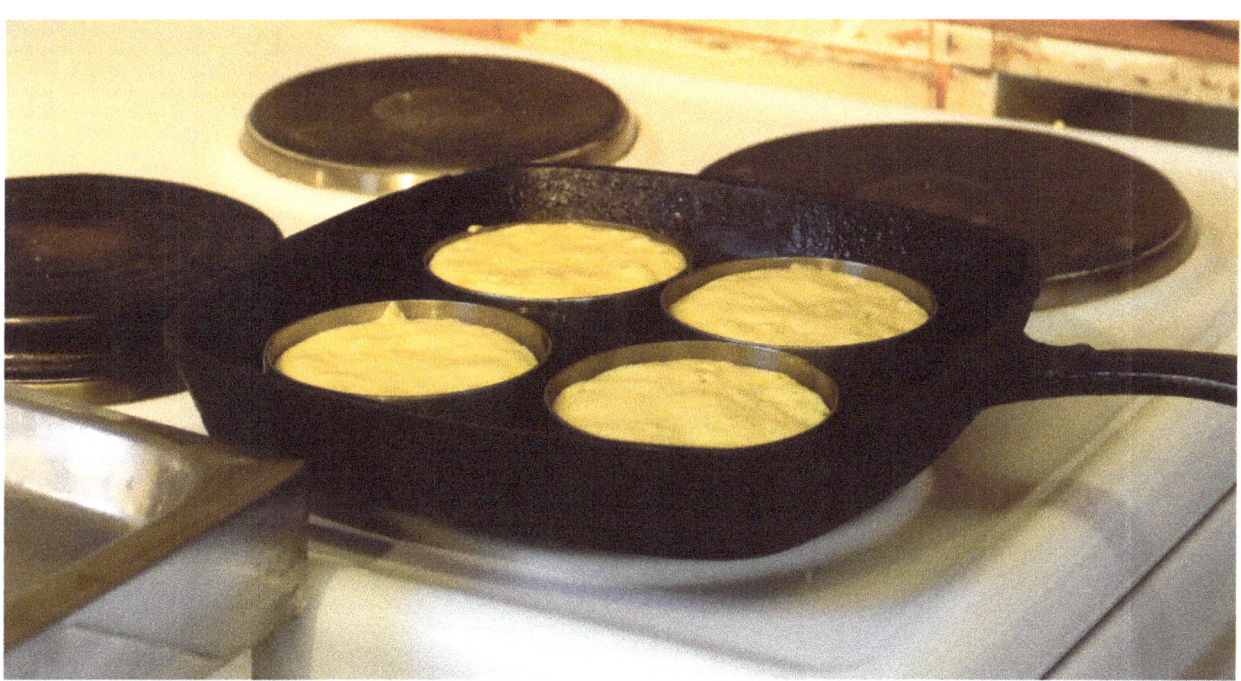

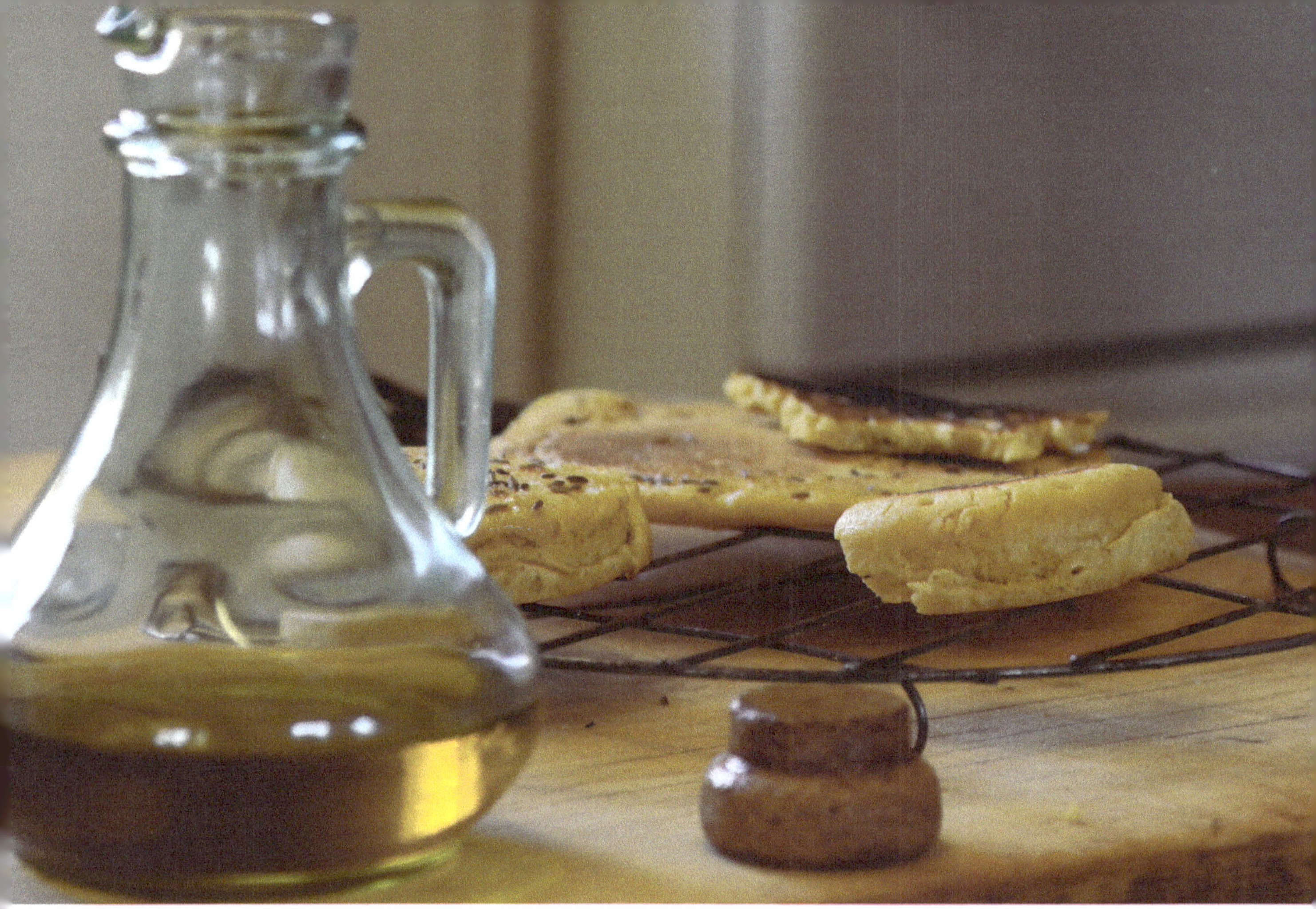

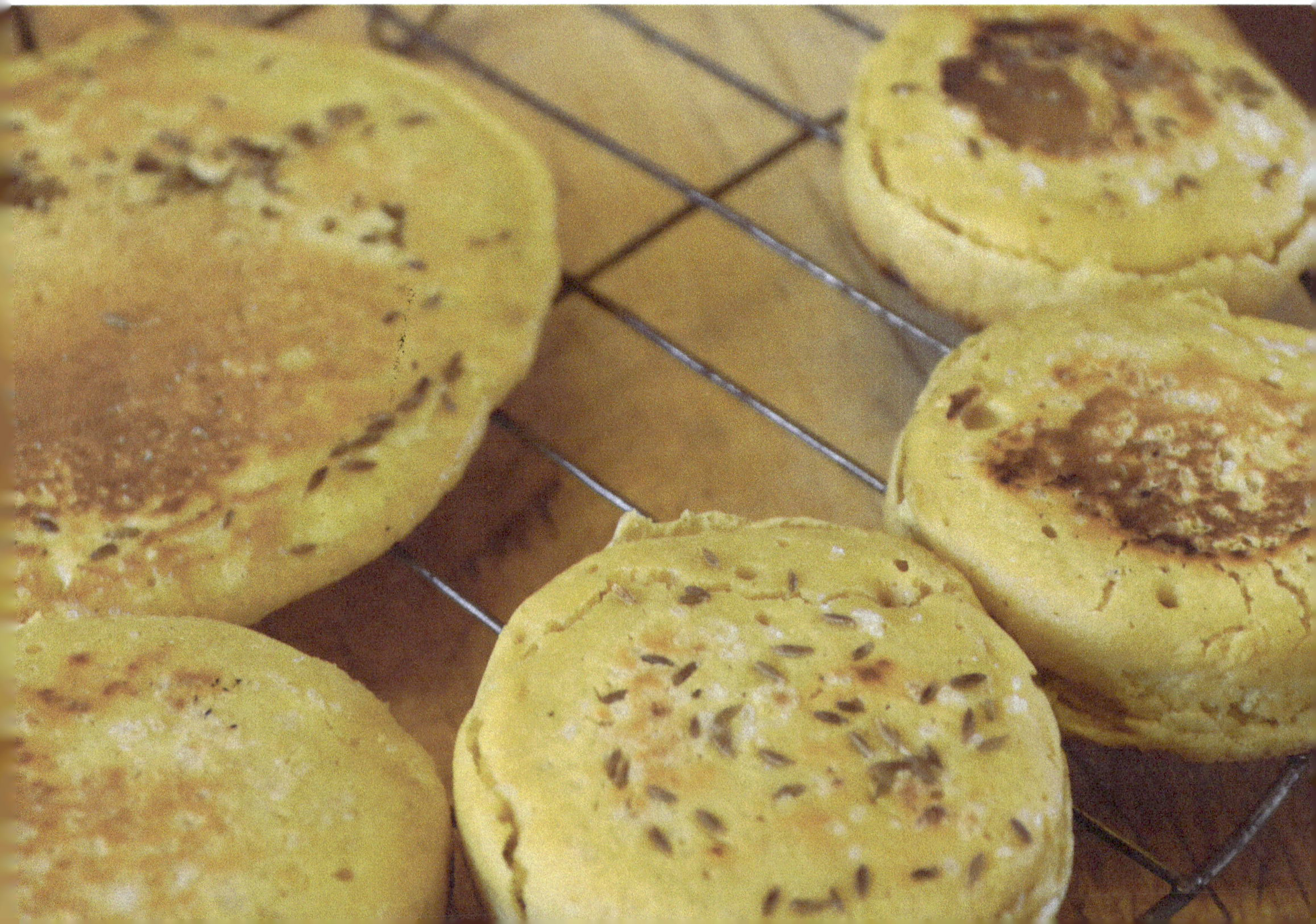

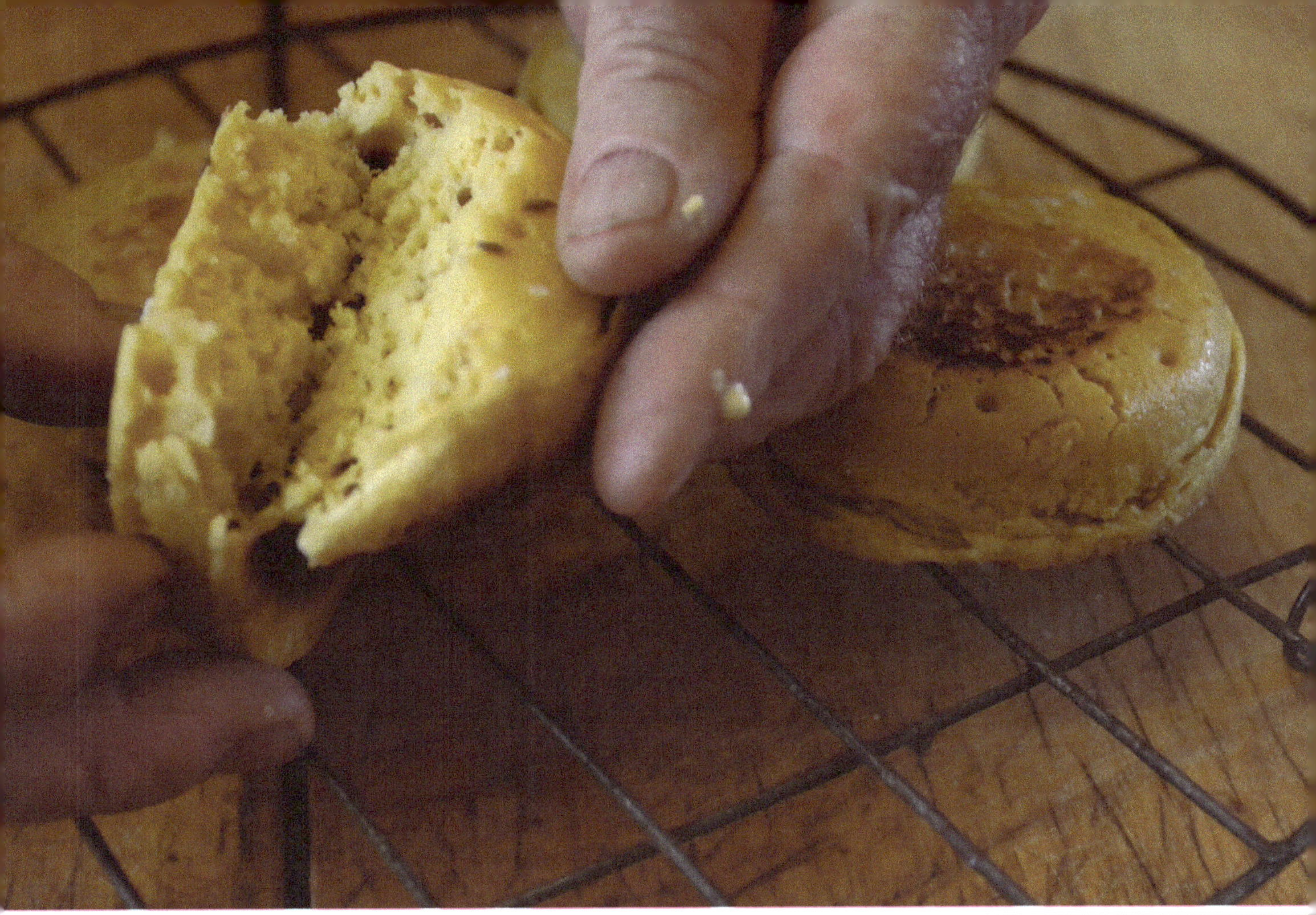

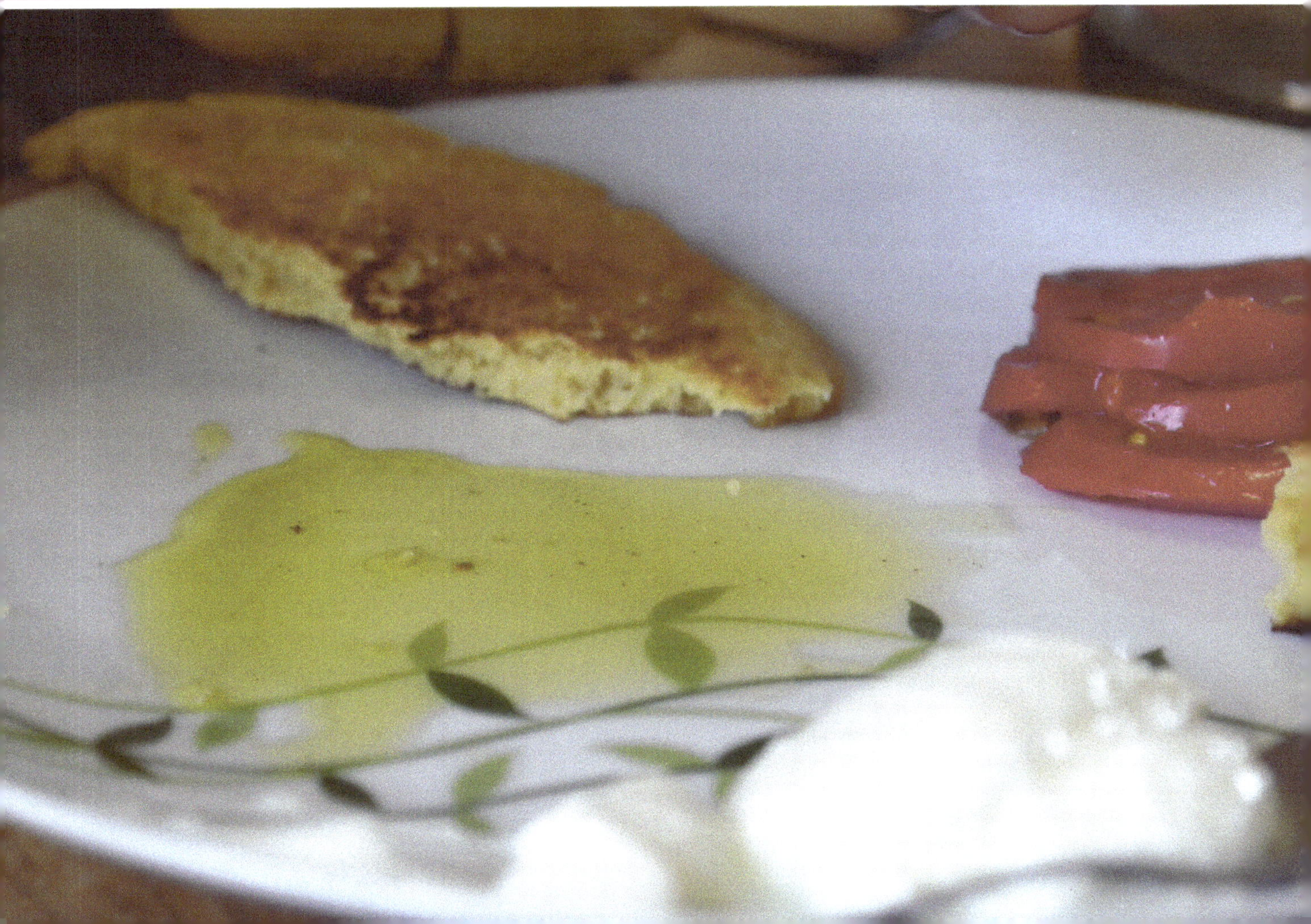

BARLEY AND OAT RING BREADS

Ingredients:

- 150 g barley or oat meal.
- 150 g warm water.
- 2 tbsp seed starter.
- ¼ tsp bicarb soda.
- ½ tsp sea salt.
- 2 tbsp warm water.

(Milk or plant milks may be used instead of water)

The best oatmeal to use is "pinhead" which has few particles larger than a pinhead as well as finer floury particles. The barley meal should be the same, or a little coarser.

Barley grain is usually available in supermarkets or in good food stores as "pearled barley". Grind it in a coffee grinder for the best results if suitable barley meal is not available. These may also be made with either (roasted) buckwheat, emmer wheat, regular wheat and probably other cereals. This makes 4 nice rounds.

Method

Mix the barley or oatmeal, 150 g water and seed leaven. Make into a batter, cover and leave 12 hours or overnight until risen and active. This will dry up to some extent as the meal absorbs water.

Sprinkle the salt on the batter, dissolve the soda in the warm water and gently stir in to the batter until well mixed and smooth. Cover and leave for 5 minutes to activate.

This is the batter for ring breads. To make a large pan bread (pancake) as is traditional, add an extra 2 tablespoons of water (whole milk or plant milk if preferred) to the above mix.

Heat a griddle to medium and lightly oil or brush with butter or ghee. Brush the inside of the rings with good oil (cold-pressed) or butter. When the griddle is ready, place the rings on to warm up briefly and ladle batter to a bit more than half way up the ring. Turn the heat down a little, the heat of the griddle should not be fierce or these will burn, better to err on the cooler side.

The batter will rise slowly, fill the ring and be nicely holey. It will slowly set and be ready to flip after 5 minutes. When the batter starts to separate from the ring, so slip a knife around the bread to release it. Flip it over and toast the other side for 2 minutes or more for toast lovers.

If the griddle or fry-pan has a lid, these are improved in volume by covering for the first few minutes with the lid to create some steaminess.

If making a pan bread with the extra-thinned batter, pour a cupful onto the hot griddle and swirl or spread to make a large thin 30cm diameter "pancake". It should splatter a bit and be very lacey or holey with bubbles rising and breaking the surface, and thin enough not to need flipping, but cooking both sides may suit. This may also be made a bit thicker and more substantial and can be finished under a grill.

WHEAT RING BREADS AND CRUMPETS

The same sort of bread may be made with wheat flour as well, and this is worth doing with any excess leaven. Essentially, this is simply baking the leaven and is a no-fuss way of making breads or crumpets.

Use any of the leavens when mature and peaking, rather than old and tired, add soda dissolved in a little water, add salt, rest briefly and pour into rings in the same way. A thinner batter will make excellent instant crumpets or a thicker one, more bready rounds. This has to be the simplest way to make sourdough bread. Adding the soda is optional, the ring breads will be rustic and a little twangy in flavour.

BARLEY AND HAZELNUT RING BREAD

Griddle breads are traditional with nut meal stirred into the final batter at the same time as the soda is added.

Roast hazelnuts, grind or crush them and add 2-3 tbsps, (about 30 g) to the batter.

Alternatively, add other toasted or un-toasted nuts: walnuts or almonds, pistachio or pine nuts. Use 20g of chestnut flour in the initial batter as a substitute for some of the barley or oat meal to make barley, oat and chestnut ring breads ... to be served at Rivendell no doubt!

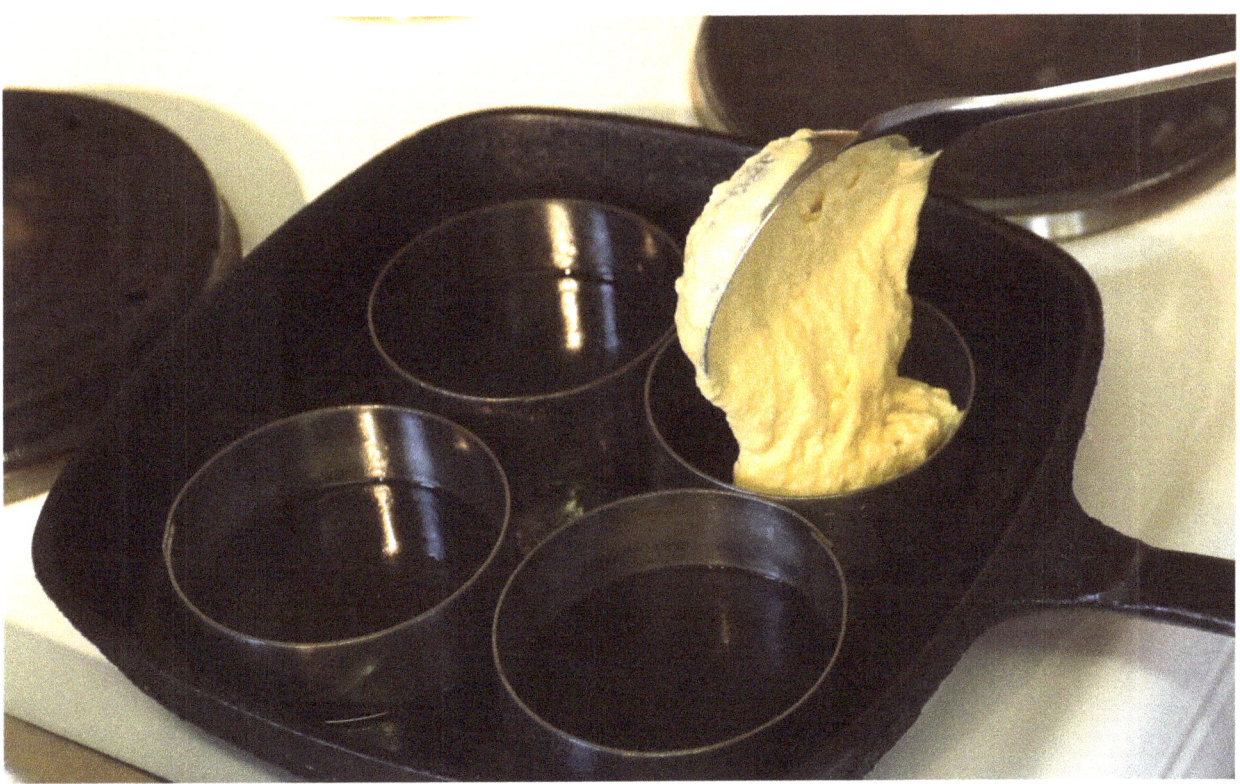

The Sourdough Loaf

FINALE RING BREAD
Uni Appam.

Ingredients:
- 1 cup Indica rice - either idli rice or basmati (preferably brown basmati).
- 1 ½ cups water.
- 1 cup palm sugar.
- 2 medium-size very ripe bananas, mashed (not pureed).
- 1 tsp ground cardamom.
- 2 tbsp seed leaven.

There are a few forms of appam, but mostly they are little globes of deep-fried sourdough, sweet cakes made in the south of India. Usually appam are made in a specially indented fry pan. As these are not common, I found the delicious appam can be made as the finale of the ring breads, in the rings as above. Failing this, make them as a pancake.

Appam are easy to make and delectable, really worth adding to a culinary repertoire, a glimpse of the dizzying range of foods which are made with sourdough.

In the ambient (27°C) heat of Kerala, these ferment readily overnight. I have added seed starter to help them on their way in cooler climes, and this works perfectly, but the batters must be kept warm.

Method

Soak the rice overnight or 8 hours. Drain and puree to a gritty, not smooth batter with 1 cup, or a little more depending on the rice, of the soaking water.

Add the rest of the ingredients, mix well until smooth, cover, keep warm and leave for 8-12 hours or overnight.

The batter should be frothy and well-risen. Spoon into rings using a little more oil or ghee than with the other ring breads. Bicarb may be added if desired, 1/2 tsp in 1 tbsp water gently mixed in to the batter, to make a lighter cake.

These appam will scorch colourfully on the bottom which adds to the flavour.

Whole cane sugar may be used, rapidura, panella or Indian gur. If the palm sugar is hard, add a little very hot water to soften it to a damp mass.

BUCKWHEAT AND CHESTNUT RING BREADS

Ingredients:
- 130 g (toasted) buckwheat meal.
- 20 g chestnut flour.
- 240 g warm water.
- 2 tbsp seed leaven.
- ½ tsp sea salt.

Almost the best of these is the buckwheat and chestnut ring bread. Harking to traditional roots, both buckwheat and chestnuts are important foods, and "polenta" was usually made from one of these (or millet or chickpeas) as a staple before maize supplanted them.

Buckwheat, as in the kasha of the Slavs, needs to be lightly toasted in a pan or the oven before use, otherwise the taste is not appealing. Toasted until it is "nutty" and reddish in colour, it can be stored, ready for use. Grind the toasted buckwheat to a gritty or sandy meal, not a flour.

Method
Make a batter with the buckwheat meal and chestnut flour, and stir in the seed leaven. Keep warm and this will ferment overnight (8 hrs) or a little longer.

Add salt and stir gently without deflating to create a uniform texture, and leave to rest 5 minutes. Ladle into oiled rings, half way up the ring on the griddle or pan and cook as for the other ring breads.

An option is to dissolve ¼ tsp of bicarb soda in 1 tbsp of warm water, and gently stir in to the batter with the salt. Leave for 5 minutes then proceed as for other ring breads. This version is lighter, more aerated, but both versions admirably perform the function of a "burger" bun.

SAFFRON OATCAKES

When the initial oat batter is being made, measure out the water to be mixed with the soda and add a good pinch of saffron. Leave to steep overnight.

After 12 hours, dissolve the soda in the saffron water and add to the batter with sea salt. Stir it gently until well-mixed and leave to recover for 5 minutes. Griddle as above. Excellent with salmon, sweet butter and proper cider.

MUFFYNS

...Or "English muffins" are made in the same way as the ring breads, on a griddle, but the ring is not used, as these are made from a bread dough. Again, bicarb soda may be added for extra aeration and a milder flavour.

The dough process is the same as in traditional sourdough recipes, and most of the doughs here are suitable for griddle cooking. The brown crusty dough (p 93) made from sifted stoneground wholemeal is ideal, but the wholemeal (p 97) and white (p 91) are also excellent and for a difference, the purple wheat and yellow corn dough (p 135). It is simply a tack, a change of technique. Why not use some dough for a loaf and the rest for a few griddle brads?

Method
When the dough has had its initial proof, 1 hour for wholemeal, 2 hours for white, leave it for another ½ hour, and break off a few 100 g pieces, or convert the whole dough, dust hands with flour and roll them into rounds with as few fissures as you can manage. Cover with a cloth and plastic and let relax for 30 minutes. After the rest, re-round them, relax for 2 minutes and slowly flatten each to a round. Dust the surface lightly with flour as needed. Cover them again for 15 minutes and then turn them over to flatten the upper-side, letting gravity do the work.

Brush the griddle lightly with good oil or ghee and use medium heat. When it is hot, poke each cake with a fork a few times and place on the griddle. They will start to rise and toasty aromas will waft. Turn the heat down to about ¼ as the cakes are placed on the griddle. Cook them for 4-5 minutes and then flip over and griddle the other side for 4 minutes. Remove and allow to cool on a cooling wire. When these are still warm they are customarily split around the side with the thumbs, and opened to receive slabs of butter.

Making griddle breads like this is really convenient and the small round cake or bread is ideal for lunches or split and grilled with cheese or eaten with soups, stews or salads.

An option is to chop up the dough after it has had an initial proof, and re-mix it by hand lightly with ½ teaspoon of bicarb soda dissolved in a tablespoon or two of warm water. This doesn't require much mixing. Leave it to relax for 5 minutes, then proceed to divide and shape. These require much less proof and aeration is increased. Give them a few minutes to relax after being shaped into rounds, then flip them over so both sides will be flattened, relax a few minutes and griddle them.

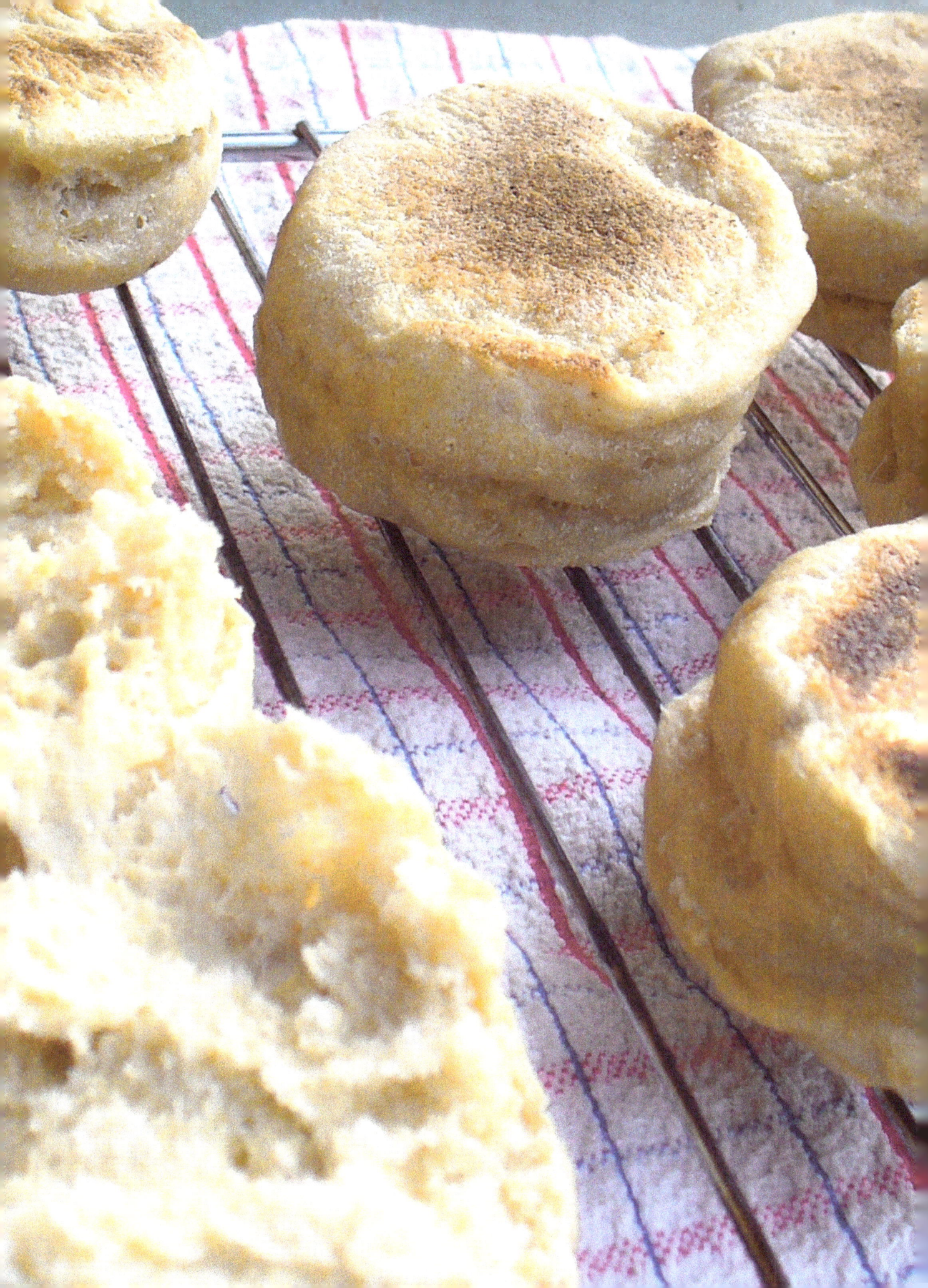

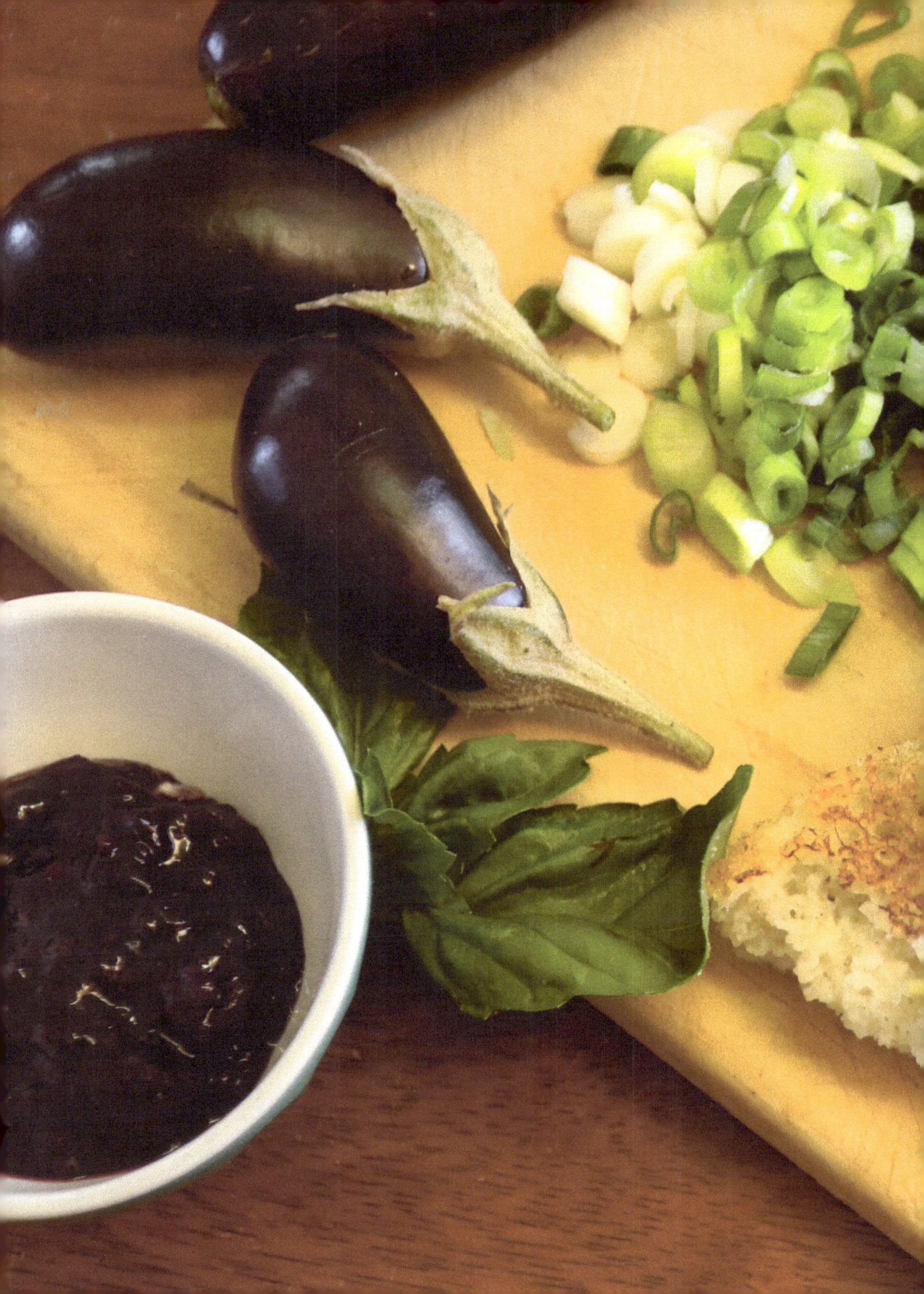

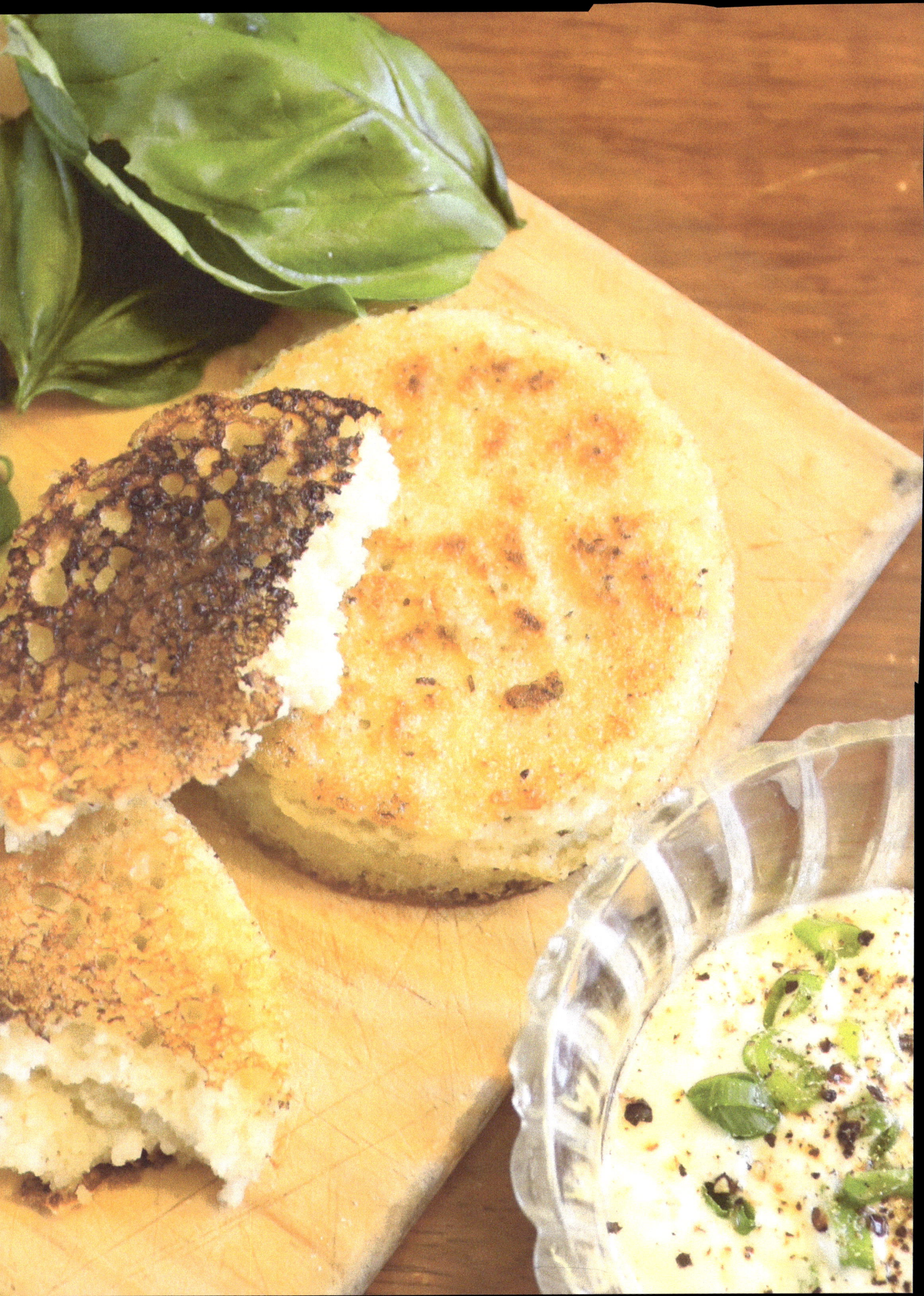

SOCCA: CHICKPEA MANNA

Ingredients.

- 200 g chickpea flour (besan).
- 220 g water.
- 1 heaped tsp of sea salt.
- 2 tsp stock leaven.
- 1 or 2 tsp cumin seeds.
- 2 tbsp extra-virgin olive oil.

That socca has a different name in many Mediterranean ports attests to its great antiquity. Socca is a chickpea-flour flatbread of varying thickness and style, but even if the names vary all its variations are made from the same ingredients, chickpea flour, water, salt and extra-virgin olive oil, and usually, cumin seeds.

It is "fundamental mode" for bread making, being simply mixed and baked, the original pancake, the simplest and easiest way to make a bread. Of very modern importance is that all of these chickpea goodies are ancient jewels re-discovered as gluten-free on a culinary "antiques road-show", to soothe your modern tummy. I would prefer to eat these gems than a contrived gluten-free bread which just looks like bread but does not deliver the promise.

Chickpeas are as old as civilisation, and then some. Similar breads to socca are made right around the " Med rim" through west Asia and down to Gujarat in India, where dhokla is important, a simple ferment of chickpeas.

This follows the ancient trade routes of the Indus civilisation and later the Roman spice trade routes. Socca-type dishes are probably the original method of using chickpeas as food and the fact they are all coastal or sea-port specialities demonstrates the significance of trade to gastronomy.

Most commentators refer to socca and its cousins as being "unfermented" but this refers both to a current incarnation, and to the fact that it is a recipe minus its context. As I have mentioned, the batter of chickpeas ferments rapidly as soon as it is made, especially because it is a child of warmer climes. Simply having it at hand in a commercial situation, in a hot climate, that is, to keep serving hungry customers, would cause it to ferment rapidly, resulting in a much nicer flavour and texture.

In an old Italian reference to socca/farinata/cecina the writer opined that the dish was much better when the batter was " left in the sun all day", that is to ferment and gain some aeration and lightness, with the increased digestibility (from the fermentation) not lost on the eaters. Others simply state in their methodology that socca is at its best when the batter is left to stand for a few hours.

One ancient link is the curious use of cumin seed in some socca, with cumin not at all common in Italian or southern French food. Cumin seed is used on Gujarati dhokla and again we see the direct spice trade of old, from Gujarat and Kerala to Genoa and ports such as Nice.

Taking my lead from this global perspective, and giving the recipe a context beyond ingredients, I have found chickpea flour to ferment actively

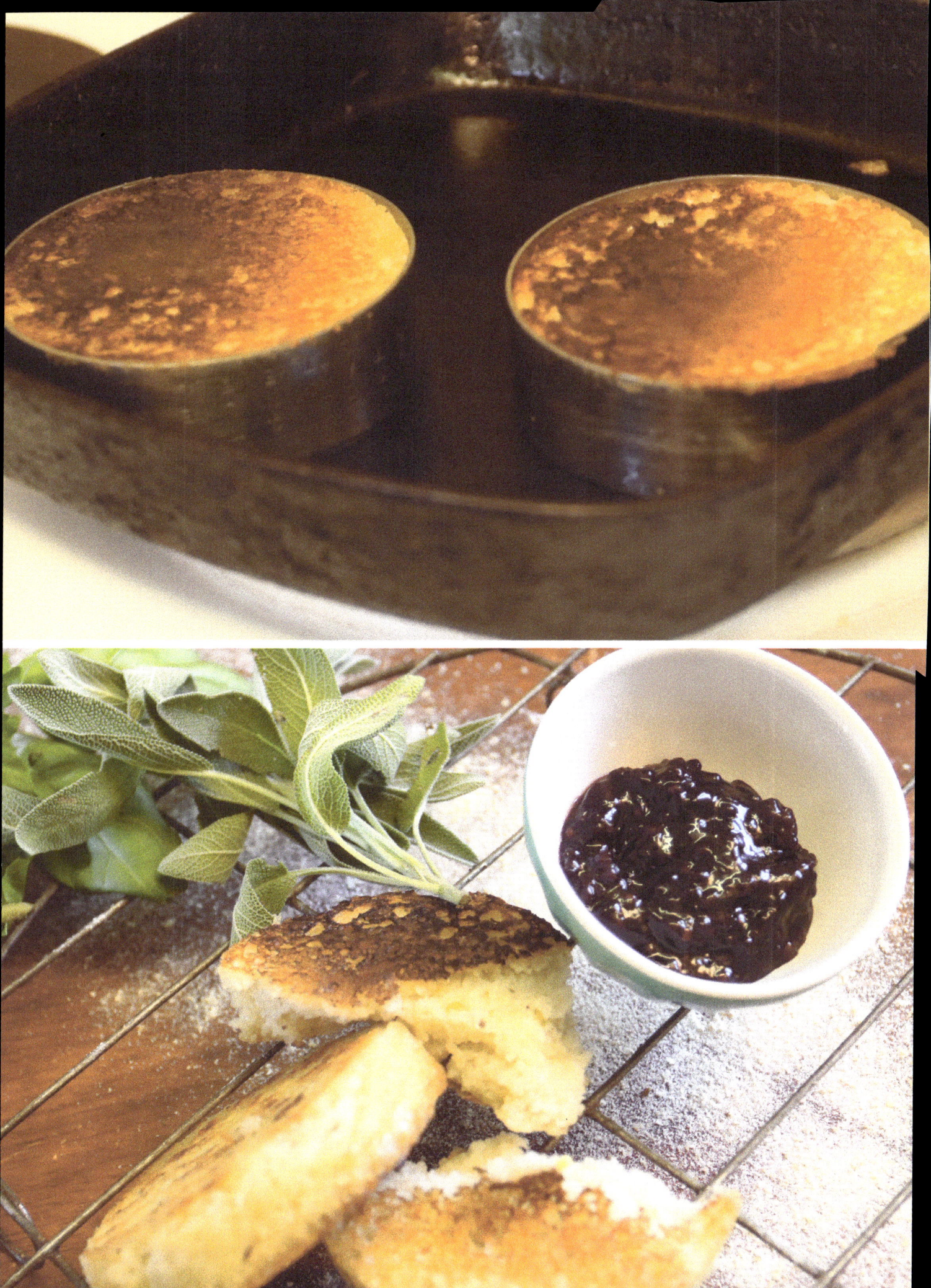

and the ferment to enhance the flavour noticeably as well as assist digestibility.

Method (for unfermented Socca)
To make unfermented socca, simply mix chickpea flour, water and salt to a thick batter, swirling in some extra-vigin olive oil. This is spread on a pan, strewn with cumin seeds and baked in a wood-fired oven at high heat. The baking is rapid and the socca an important "snack" often accompanied by a sweet wine.

It may also be made in a fry-pan with plenty of extra-virgin olive oil, like a large pancake, and it is equally delicious and easy if there is no hot brick oven available.

Taking it further, if the batter is made a little thicker or stiffer and dropped onto the hotplate, it emerges as a colourful crispy fritter of great flavour when salted.

The batter may also be griddled in an oiled crumpet ring which makes a delightful well-risen yellow socca-cake or little round ring bread which is superb with a meal or as a snack. The flavour is reminiscent of a mild cheese and the texture slightly dry, the perfect foil for a tasty sauce or with fruit chutney and curd….or a glass of sweet wine.

When the batter is allowed to ferment, or purposely fermented by adding some stock leaven, the dish is much improved. In a warm climate or summer, the batter is easily fermented by leaving it to stand overnight or for at least 8 hours, in which time it will "turn".

Method (for fermented Socca)
Either simply mix the ingredients minus the stock leaven and leave to turn overnight (in hot weather) or add the stock leaven if it is cooler. When ready, the batter will show aeration if un-seeded or quite an active ferment if seeded with the stock leaven. I have had the batter fermented within a few hours from adding the stock leaven… made in the afternoon and ready to accompany dinner the same night.

When the batter is ready, gently mix in a tablespoon of extra-virgin olive oil and a teaspoon of salt.

Heat extra-virgin olive oil in a pan over medium heat and add the cumin seeds. Let them fry briefly and add the batter. It will quickly spread and may be assisted to spread with a wooden spoon.

Small holes will break the surface and when these are a-plenty, flip the socca and cook the other side for a minute. Nice red colours appear to contrast the rich yellow centre. Drain on paper or a wire, sprinkle with good salt and enjoy while hot.

To make the fritters or socca cakes, make the batter thicker, "dropping" from a spoon. Toast the cumin seeds lightly and gently stir in to the batter. Oil the crumpet ring well and place in the hot pan, turn the heat down to about 1/3. Drop in the batter until half way up the ring, it should rapidly spread and aerate nicely. Cook for 4-5 minutes and flip for another 2 minutes. After about 3 minutes the ring can be removed, clearing the edge from the ring with a knife.

Even more delicious, roast 3 tbsp of pine nuts lightly crush them and gently add 3 tbsp to the batter, resting for 5 minutes before cooking.

If you have a hot oven handy, the socca may be thinly spread in a well-oiled pan (with extra-virgin olive oil) and baked. This will be done in 3-5 minutes.

In the same way as the ring breads, bicarb soda may be added with a little water to increase aeration and sweeten the flavour.

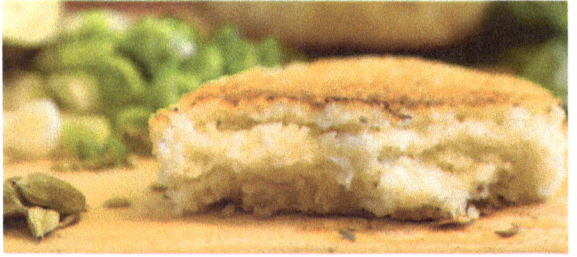

DHOKLA
Indian chickpea sourdough bread.

Kaman dhokla, is essentially the same as the socca, except it is steamed. There are many varieties of Gujarati dhokla, all traditionally fermented and steamed, much in the manner of idli (p 163). In this recipe, you will require a tray that can comfortably fit inside a larger pan for steaming.

Dhokla is often made as "instant" by using bi-carb soda or eno fruit salts as the leavening agent, and not fermented at all. There is even a dhokla-western "roti" bread substitution, diamonds of fluffy white bread with the traditional dhokla accompaniments, neatly demonstrating the place of dhokla as "bread" within Indian culinary culture.

Dhokla batter is poured into an oiled tray and steamed as a block. When cool it is cut into squares or diamonds, and often any or a combination of black mustards seeds, kalonji (nigella) or cumin are quickly fried in virgin sesame coconut or mustard oil and the tasty hot oil is tipped on the dhokla It is also often dressed with chopped fresh coriander, and often fresh crushed ginger and chopped green chillies, which are are stirred into the batter before steaming. Coriander, tamarind or mint chutney is usually served with dhokla as well.

Method
To make dhokla, follow the directions for socca, perhaps doubling the recipe so the dhokla is about 3cm thick and pour into the tray. Place a few cups of water into a deep pan over medium heat, and when steam starts to emanate, place the dhokla tray in the pan on a small stand or inverted bowl. Cover the container with a lid and let it steam for 12 to 15 minutes. Put a cotton tea-towel under the steamer lid to make sure no condensed steam drips back on to the dhokla.

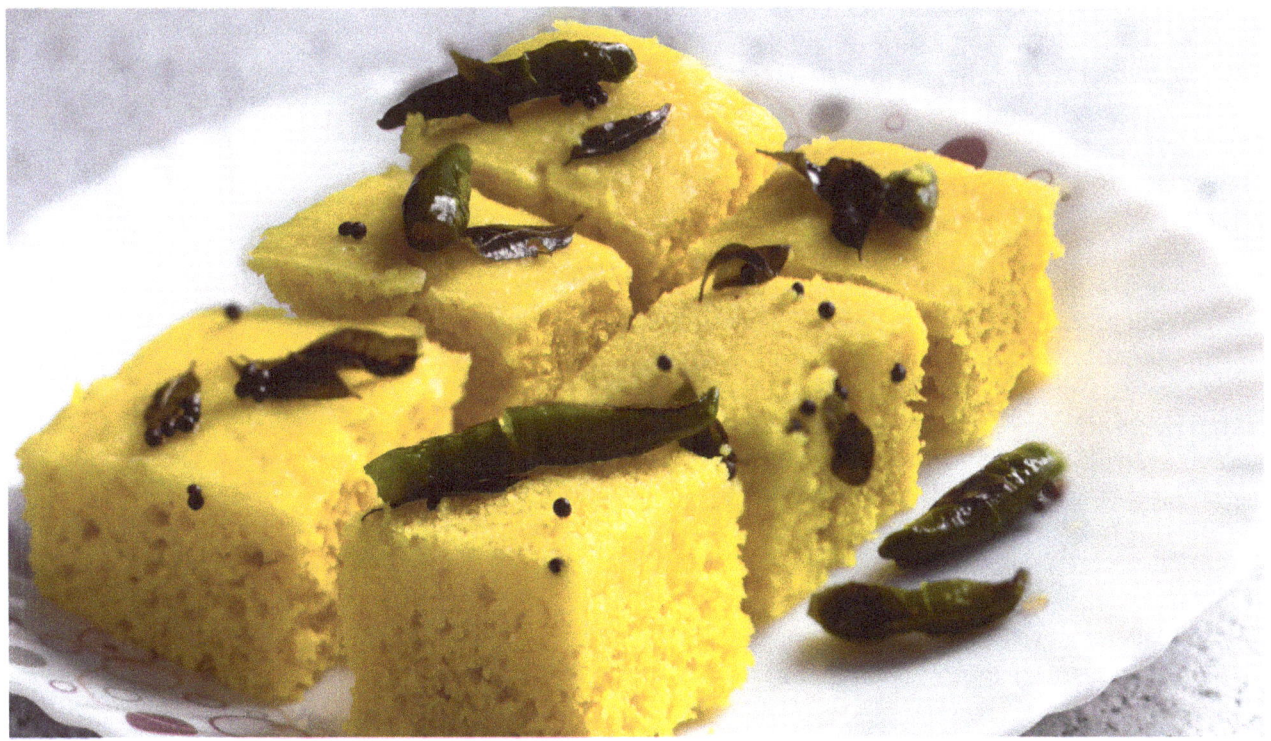

IDLI

Indian sourdough.

Ingredients.

Idli:
- 2 cups rice.
- ½ - 1 cup urid dal (also known as brown or black gram or urad bean).
- ½ tablespoon of fenugreek seeds if desired.
- Water to cover.

A chutni for idli:
- 1 cup coriander leaves.
- 1 cup grated coconut (fresh or frozen) but not desiccated.
- 1 green chilli chopped.
- 1 x 5 cm piece of fresh ginger.
- 1 tsp of lemon or lime juice.
- 1 tbsp of palm sugar or whole-juice cane sugar (rapidura or panella).
- 2 tsp of salt.
- 2 tbsp of virgin sesame, coconut or mustard oil.
- 1 tsp of black mustard seeds.
- A big pinch of curry leaves.

These are small white-ish sourdough cakes or breads made from rice and dal. Originating in the south of India, they are enjoyed everywhere on the sub-continent today, and well they may be. I was overwhelmed and overjoyed to "discover" these in India many years ago while wandering the streets in search of gold. I found it.

If you live in a cold-cool clime, probably just wonder about them as they require a consistently warm climate to work well…..or use a warming cabinet or bain-marie, but they are often not quite as tasty. As with dhokla, there are analogs made with baking powder or bicarb soda, even "fruit salts", but again they are far from the original as the flavour and nutrition are compromised.

The flavour is mildly sour, as with a good sourdough, tempered by the sweetness of rice and the typical taste of the legume dal. The texture is a wonder, light and fluffy almost like good white bread! As these are eaten with, usually, coconut-coriander chutney as well as a masala of some kind, the flavours synergise to delight, especially at breakfast. They are also excellent with good butter and other more western flavours, even eggs.

This is a tropical sourdough and is more in keeping with a hot climate as the spontaneous fermentation processes are inherently "natural". Being steamed in 10 minutes, rather than baked for some time, with attendant oven heating and racing ferments, they are warm climate-appropriate. Baking often seems like over-kill in the warmer and sub-tropical or tropical zones, and may even be too "heating" for the body.

Idli are also resource-friendly in that steaming uses up much less energy than baking, and hundreds may be steamed on a small clay stove fuelled only with dried grass and grass stems.

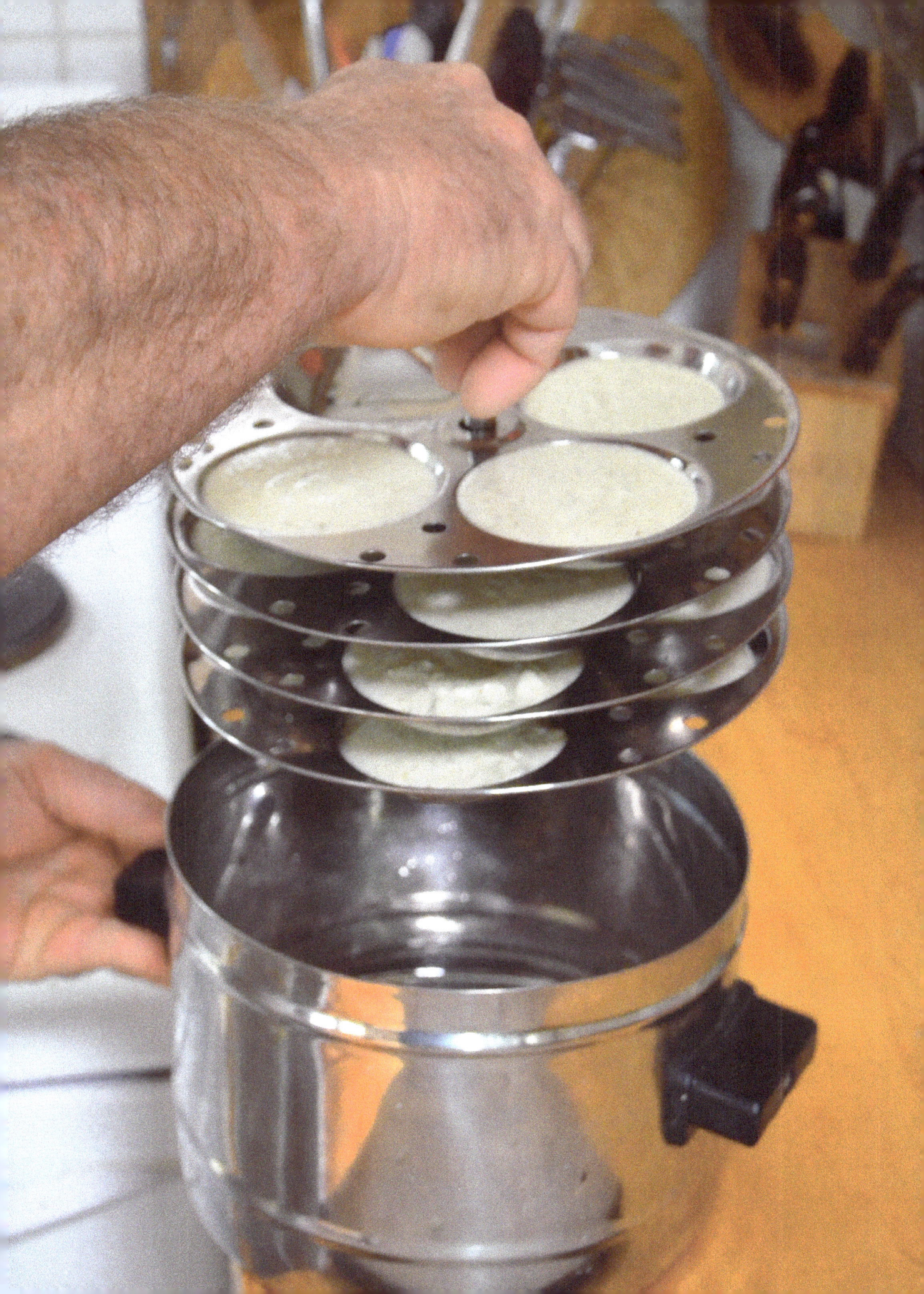

We have traditionally observed the maxims of nature in food, and Idli are a perfect example of the reality of "local", as we perceive the difference between this sourdough and a crusty French bread. Wheat does not grow in the south of India and rice does not grow in the cooler climates, yet sourdough is the master in both, the culture of cultures.

Nutritionally, idli are a masterpiece as the combination of rice and dal meshes the proteins, providing more protien and a more balanced form of protein, as do wheat and chickpeas which are more the staple of west-Asia and the Mediterranean. Besides the protein being balanced, the fermentation unlocks minerals and creates more nutrients such as vitamins, in the same way as a conventional Western European sourdough. And in addition to all of this, idli are gluten-free and easy to digest, which is also perfect in the heat of the tropics.

What makes idli even more desirable in a warm climate is that they are so easy to make. One does not fuss over the sourdough starter. The method is to soak black gram also known as urid dal overnight, and at the same time the rice is soaked. In the south of India, the rice is specifically called "idli rice" and is a small pearly grain. Then the two are ground and combined and allowed to ferment. This happens rapidly and a surprisingly foamy mix rises to double the volume.

The ferment is then simply spooned into an idli steamer, which consists of small cups suspended on a central stem and sealed. A well-known and easily available egg-poacher does this well, so no need to search for an idli steamer, although you will as soon as you become familiar with these wonderful breads.

Idli rice from the Indian grocer works perfectly. If this is not available, use basmati or other "Indica" rice (usually long grain). If using "Japonica" rice, or brown rice, parboil for 3 minutes first, drain then allow to cool. Other dal may be substituted such as mung and even channa (chickpeas) which makes them accessible and easy.

Usually skinned dal are used, but often an idli maker (walla) will use unhulled black dal which gives the idli a grey hue, and more flavour. One idli walla I haunted in Varanasi also soaked fenugreek seeds with the dal and another added onion. I have also seen them with ginger and grated carrot in the mix.

In Karnataka, rava idli are made with suji (coarse semolina) instead of rice, and usually leavened with soda. Wheat sourdough may be used, as per the ring bread recipes, and steamed in the same way.

One secret is to ensure the rice and dal mix is not ground too finely. The mix should be slightly gritty to feel. This prevents the idli being gluggy. Once the ferment is completed it will hold for a day or so and even longer if refrigerated and brought back to room temperature before steaming.

Any left-over idli batter can be thinned with water or coconut water, and spread on a griddle to make the even more famous south Indian speciality, dosa. These are perfect for lunch, after breakfast idli. They are made from the same mix, but are crunchy and appetising, usually served with turmeric-laced aloo (potato) masala. Dosa are similar to the Mediterranean speciality socca, demonstrating the universality of technique made local.

Method for Idli

Soak rice and dal separately overnight for 8 hours, with plenty of water on the dal. Strain and reserve the soaking water from the dal.

Wet-grind both separately to a paste, not too fine, it should feel a little gritty. Use the dal water to grind them both. When adding the soaking water, the batter should be more thick than thin. If in doubt err on the side of a thicker batter. Mix both together, add half a tablespoon of sea-salt, which keeps the ferment "clean".

Cover with a cloth and leave to ferment. In India this happens overnight. Some idli wallas add a little of the previous day's batter to accelerate the process. If you are in a hot climate, especially if it is humid, or in summer, it will happen naturally.

When the batter is frothy and active, spoon into the oiled, or ghee'd cups until just level. Steam over high heat for 10-12 minutes. Wet your finger and touch the top of one, if it sticks, steam more, if the finger does not stick, they are ready.

Turn out on a cooling wire rack.

Some makers line the idli steamer cups with cheese cloth and when a large steamer is used with about 50 cups, these are turned out dramatically amid copious steam, which is a wonderful spectacle in the iridescent early morning bustle of India.

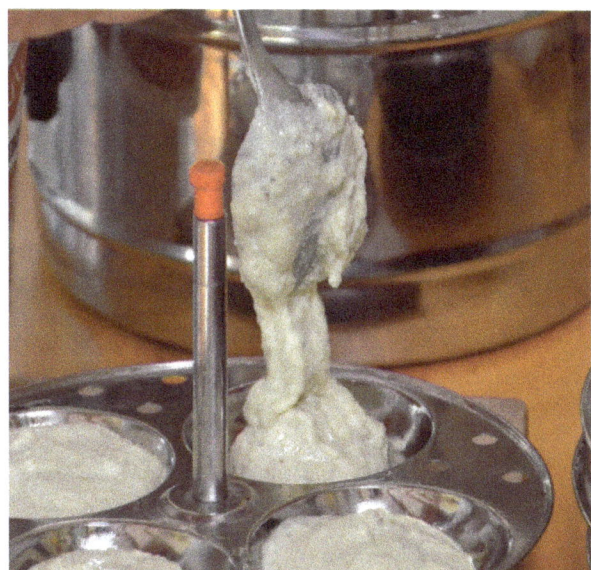

Method for chutney
Grind the coriander leaves, grated coconut, chilli, ginger, sugar and salt together and mix into the lemon or lime juice.

Heat the mustard seeds in the oil until they pop. Add the curry leaves and fry for a second longer. Mix into the chutney and enjoy with the idli.

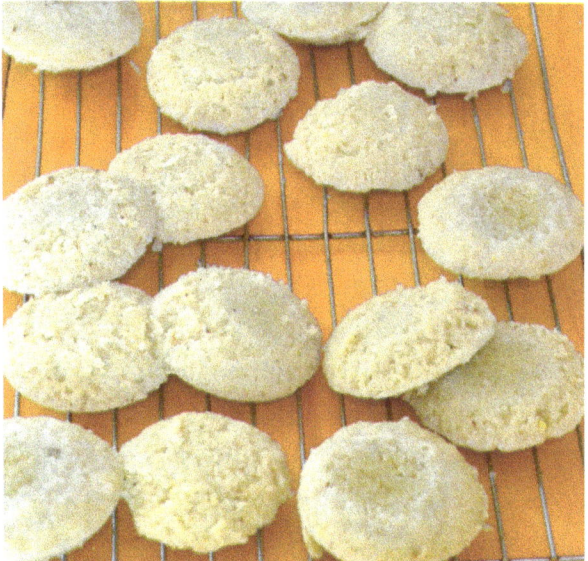

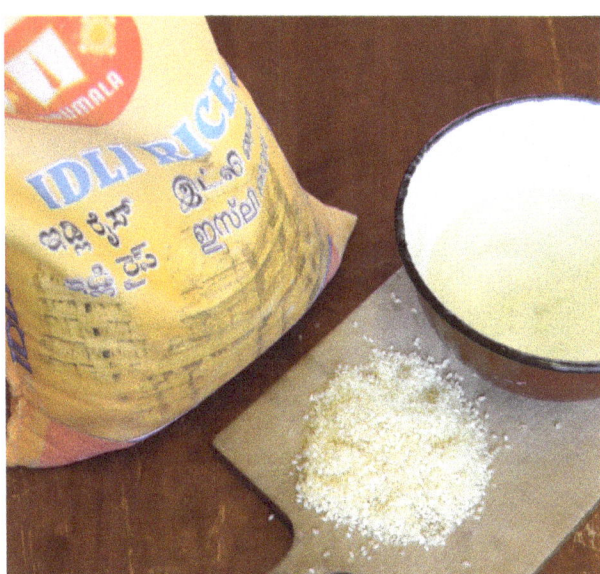

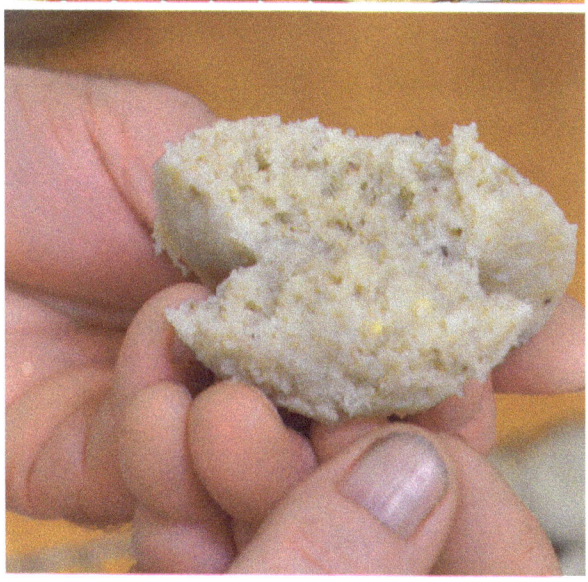

The Sourdough Loaf

SAFFRON BUNS
(of the pagan love cult.)

Ingredients.

The pre-ferment:
- 500 g organic white bread flour (wholemeal, brown or white).
- 250 g leaven.
- 275 g very warm water.

The buns:
- 8 g ginger powder.
- .8 g saffron threads - heaped (½ teaspoon, or more if you like saffron).
- ¼ tsp turmeric powder.
- 8 g ground cardamom (make from whole pods using a spice/coffee grinder).
- 5 g ground cinnamon.
- 175 g Rapidura or panella sugar.
- 125 g Saffron Milk (see method).
- 2 Eggs - 1 for buns, plus 1 for glaze.
- 75 g Butter - softened/warmed.
- 200 g Sultanas.
- 7 g Salt.
- 1 tsp Vanilla essence or scraped vanilla pods.
- 350 g extra white flour.

The glaze:
- 1 pinch saffron.
- 1 full tbsp good honey.
- 3 tbsp very hot water.
- 1 big pinch coarsely crushed fennel or caraway seeds.

The topping:
- Coarse demerara sugar

These "not cross" Oestre buns are my take on Easter. Hot cross buns can be dementing for a baker. Over the long nights making thousands upon thousands by hand, I slowly dreamt up my ideal Easter buns from scraps of history, archaeology, proto-science, contemporary accounts, pure fantasy and religion. Hot cross buns have become passe as the bastard children of industrial bakeries.

Evidently, at fertility festivals held in the before time, at lunar Easter, among other now frowned-upon activities, dough cakes, pieces...buns were baked containing aphrodisiac and narcotic/hallucinogenic herbs. Saffron is considered rasayana (rejuvenative) in India, an aphrodisiac in herbal lore, and a tradition among the Cornish in buns.

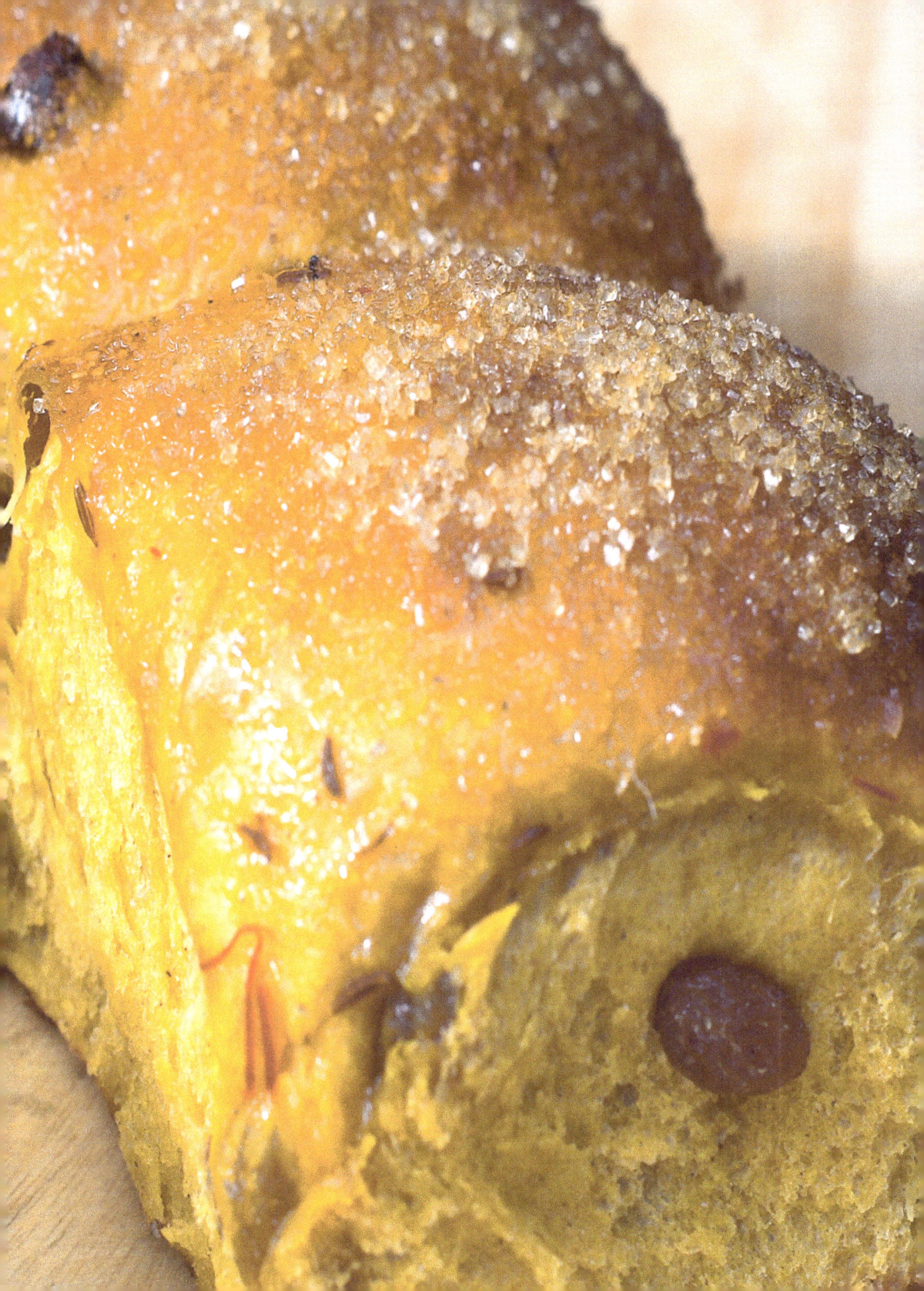

It is ancient and mysterious in flavour, unlike modern tastes, its bitterness and colour hark back to older flavour regimes and broader, challenging tastes. The other spices in the recipe are a synergy of the medieval and the orient. A friend's wife is Iranian and without a seconds thought she dubbed these "Persian hot cross buns".

The recipe is for 14-15 buns with a dough weight of 150 g, which is a substantial bun. Reduce the size to 100 g if you prefer them smaller, or alternatively treat as a "cake" and bake in a cake tin.

Because these are so good, I always double the recipe and make 28 nice sized buns which are devoured rapidly. They make a wonderful gift, or keep extraordinarily well, making legendary toast for weeks.

Traditionally, buns are made using what bakers call a "pre-ferment". This is a dough made first, before making the actual buns. It must be very active to aerate the sweet and rich dough.

Saffron is variable but ideally should be intact dark red strands. If the threads are dry and broken, they are old and not as strong, so use more.

Purchase green cardamom pods and do not remove the seeds. Using a spice grinder (coffee grinder), reduce the whole pod to a powder.

The recipe is designed for Panella or Rapidura, whole-cane-juice sugar as this adds to the overall flavour, but at least use "raw" sugar.

Vanilla essence is preferred in this recipe for a stronger flavour than pods, and use un-salted cultured butter.

Make sure to use good quality, tasty spices. The ginger powder, in particular, should not be old and flat-tasting. Fresh ginger is not suitable.

The finishing touch is to strew coarse demerara sugar crystals on the buns, finer sugar will not work

Method

The night before:
Yes this is a process...but full of meaning!
Heat the milk until near boiling and add the saffron. Cover and leave to steep, return to fridge for 10 hours, overnight or more, This can be made days in advance.

The pre-ferment:
Add leaven to the water and whisk well until frothy. Add the flour and mix to form a soft dough. Mix or knead for a few minutes until smooth and clear of lumps. Place in a bowl, cover with a tea-towel and plastic, and keep warm. After 2 hours, the dough should be well-risen and active.

The Buns:
In a bowl, cut the pre-ferment dough into a dozen pieces with a slip or knife. Add the warmed milk, the beaten egg, vanilla, sultanas, spices, salt, sugar and flour and mix well.

Add the softened butter last. Continue to mix well, this is a soft dough. When it is free of lumps, smooth and a seductive all-yellow colour, place in a bowl, cover with cloth and plastic and keep it warm (25°C). This will rise/prove for 2 hours.

When well-risen, turn out and cut into size. Weigh each piece either 150 g or 100 g. When all of the dough is divided, roll each piece in a circular motion to form balls which ideally should have a smooth-ish domed top and any creases on the bottom.

Place each piece on a tray or 2 which have been well oiled/buttered or covered with baking paper. Put each bun almost touching - kissing bakers call it, so they will rise together and when baked and cooled are gently torn apart to reveal a soft, layered "kissing crust".

Cover with cloth and plastic and keep warm for 1 hour. They should be well-risen. If not, wait a further ½ hour.

Pre heat the oven to 180°C.

Mix the reserved egg with an equal volume of water. Brush over the risen buns and bake.

After 20 minutes, the buns should have risen well and be quite dark brown on top.

The glaze:
Add the saffron to honey and very hot water. Then add the crushed fennel or caraway seeds and vanilla essence or scraped vanilla pods, and leave to steep.

The fennel/caraway seeds replicate the baroque flavour of caraway comfits…tiny caraway seeds craftily coated with sugar and once commonly strewn on buns.

Remove from the oven and turn out onto a wire cooling rack as a whole, still stuck together. Flip them on to another cooling rack dome up and without losing their heat, slap/brush on the honey glaze liberally. This will adhere and be sticky. Without hesitation, while the glaze is still hot and sticky, strew with plenty of coarse sugar crystals.

They will crackle and glisten, shimmering with goodness, the archetype of the classic bun. Well worth the effort.

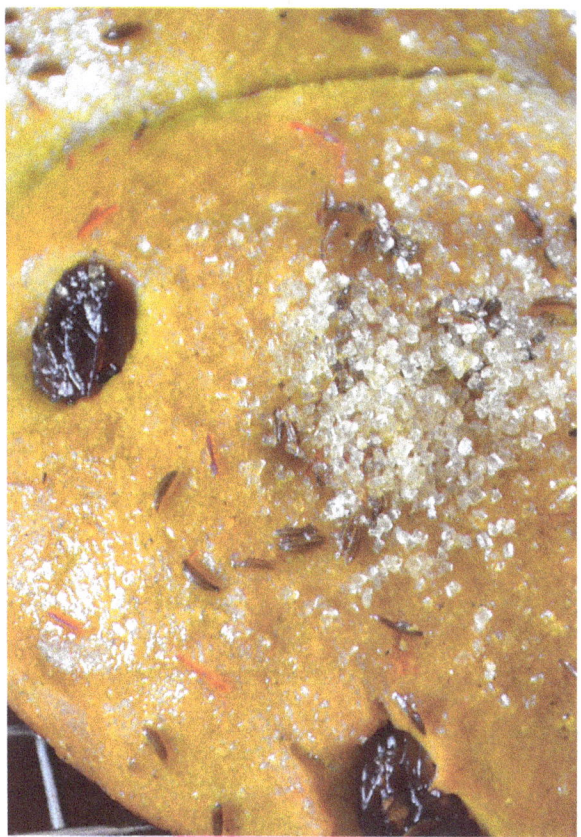

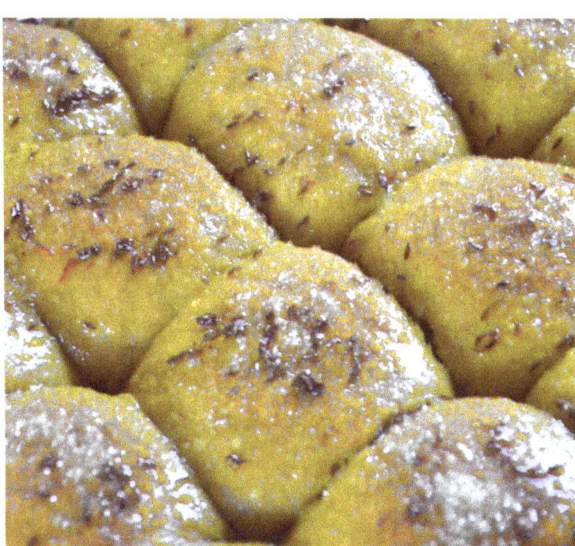

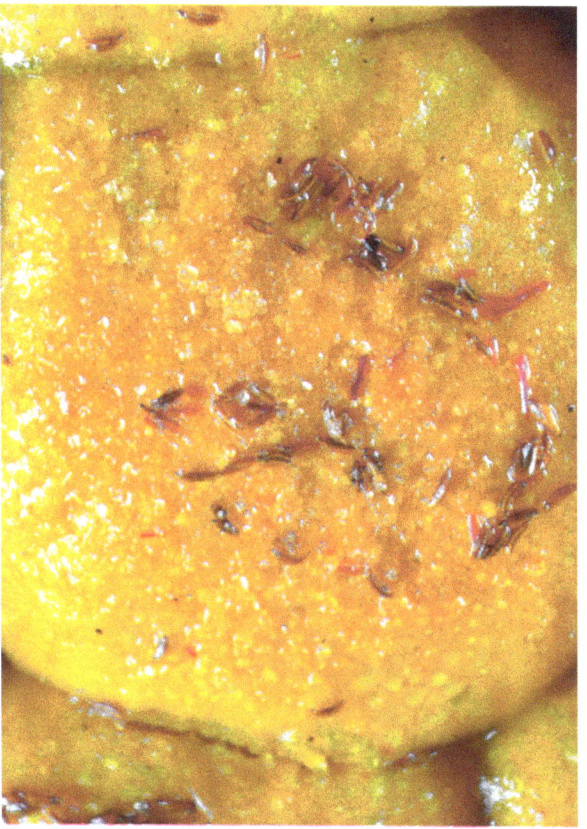

The Sourdough Loaf

STEAM BUNS

The power of food to re-kindle memories is well known. During a bread-baking class I demonstrated these steam buns, and to my dismay, discovered a middle-aged Chinese woman quietly sobbing in the shadows of the bustle. Alarmed, I went to comfort her.

These buns, made from the wholemeal dough, stirred deep memories of her childhood and a previous life which flooded in to overwhelm her. "These are exactly what I ate as a child." "This is northern Chinese bread"!

Although I was disturbed for her, a small part of me was thrilled for "getting it right", which is not easy for so much ethnic food, especially bread.

The incident also demonstrated the antiquity and universality of sourdough bread as a central and important food, far from being a trendy construct.

These buns are ideal, mid-winter with a miso and vegetable stew, "oden", or mid-summer with achar and satay chicken.

Use either the crusty white (p 91) or brown (p 93) or wholemeal (p 97) recipes after the initial proof period. The dough is divided into 75 g pieces. Roll each piece into a ball and place not touching on baking paper squares or muslin or leaves in a bamboo steamer, with any seams or joins on the bottom, and a nice domed top.

Put hot water in the wok or saucepan under the steamer and the lid on the steamer, but don't turn on the heat yet. Allow to rise for 1½ hours until well-risen, but not too much as they will drop or spread.

Turn on the heat under the steamer until boiling and steam for 10 minutes, then turn them on to a cooling rack. Using a fine spray, mist the buns with cool water briefly which creates a shiny thin skin.

This is a light, soft sourdough, without a heavy crust and makes brilliant crispy toast the next day.

Alternatively, the buns may also be filled with a tasty dry filling before being set to rise. Traditional fillings may be sweet as with azuki (redbean) jam, sweet lotus seeds, or with miso-infused vegetables or with meats, notably pork as char siu.

When the small balls of dough are formed, allow to relax for a few minutes. Then flatten these, place the filling in the centre and fold up to cover the filling, twisting to form a seal on the top which should be pinched tight to avoid leaking. Place in the steamer and proof as for un-filled buns.

STEAM BREAD

A whole loaf may be steamed instead of being baked. The three basic recipes, crusty white, crusty brown and wholemeal are suitable to steam.

Line the steamer with a moist cloth and put the dough in it to rise. Add hot water to the steamer, put the lid on and allow to prove in the same way as the bread, until well-risen. Start the water boiling and steam for 20 minutes. This produces a soft cakey loaf.

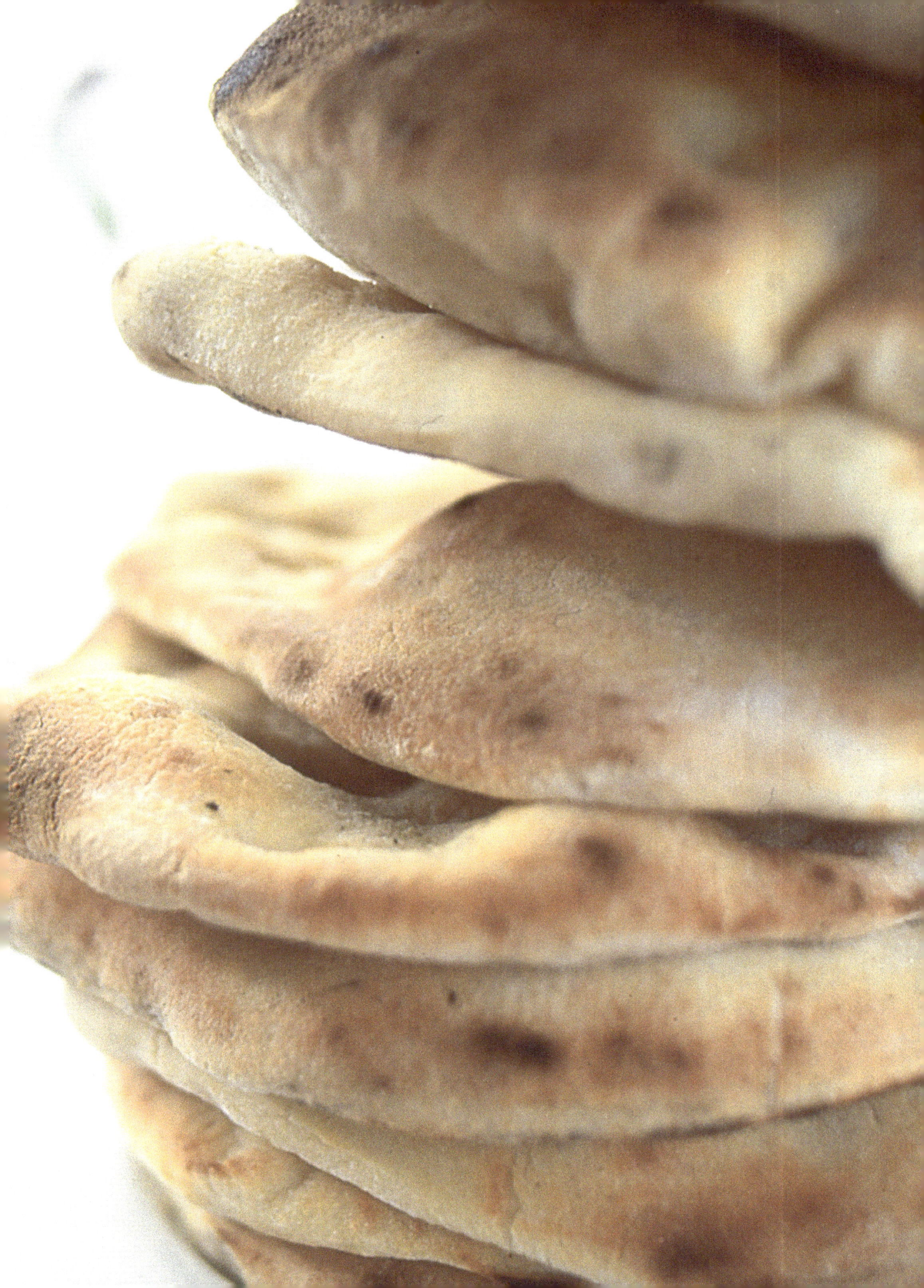

CACAO BUNS
Chocolotls.

Ingredients.

Cacao leaven:
- 120 g cacao powder.
- 200 g warm water.
- 2 tablespoons of stock leaven.

Pre-ferment:
- 250 g white bread flour.
- 125 g cacao leaven.
- 240 g warm water.
- 150 g extra white bread flour.
- 25 g cacao powder.
- 1 beaten egg.
- 40 g sweet butter or coconut butter softened or melted.
- 90 g warm whole milk (or plant milk).
- 120 g rapidura or panella sugar.
- 10 g cinnamon powder.
- 4 vanilla pods roasted and ground, or seeds scraped out, or 1- 2 tbsp best vanilla essence.

Glaze:
- 1 egg beaten with 1 tbsp of water for glazing.
- Honey or agave syrup.
- Coarse demerara sugar.

Making bread with cacao was common in the past as cacao was rightly viewed as nutritious and delicious. These buns taste like dark semi-sweet chocolate. The initial leaven is made with cacao and the fermentation brings out the deep flavours of cacao.

Recent research has indicated that chocolate is mood-altering, affecting brain chemistry, usually in a favourable way, but the research rarely states that it is cacao not chocolate which does this. Chocolate is loaded with white refined sugar, which is just junk food really, so to get the good effects of "chocolate" try cacao instead and use nutrient and flavour dense whole-juice sugars such as panella or rapidura.

Vanilla is important as a synergistic chemical and flavour to cacao. The Totonac people of Mexico first cultivated vanilla and were conquered by the Aztec largely to secure a supply of their deliciously invigorating and healthful cacao-vanilla drink for the emperor. The alkaloid in cacao is theobromine which translates as "food of the gods", and so say all of us!

Originally, vanilla pods were roasted and ground with cacao beans and this flavour is worth the effort. In the recipe it is specified to roast the vanilla and grind it. If this is too hard, roast the pods and then scrape out the seeds, but the roasting step is worthwhile.

It is worth stressing that this recipe is very temperature sensitive and the leaven, dough and rising buns must be kept warm at all stages.

Method
Mix all cacaoleaven ingredients well, cover and allow to ferment for 8 hours, after which stir well and leave another 3 hours to develop. Depending on the cacao, this may ferment vigorously or moderately, but in any case it should be noticeably active.

Warm the flour. Mix the leaven and water well and add the flour. Knead or develop it briefly, cover keep warm and leave to ferment for 2 hours.

When the pre-ferment is fully risen, chop the dough into pieces, add the cinnamon, milk, sugar, vanilla, egg and extra flour and mix well. Add the butter, mix well and knead briefly. Cover, keep warm and allow to proof for 2 hours, or a bit more until double in bulk.

Flour the surface lightly as this is sticky, and cut the dough into 100 g portions.

Roll each into a ball, using a dusting of flour and place on an oiled baking tray or on baking paper. Cover, keep warm and allow 1-1 ½ hour, or proof until double in bulk. This may take a little longer, but the buns need to be well risen.

Gently glaze with the egg-wash and bake at 180°C for 15 minutes.

As soon as the buns are out and still hot, brush with plenty of good honey or agave syrup and dredge with the sugar crystals.

A few drops of peppermint oil added to the honey or agave glaze is a worthy addition, as is 2 tablespoons of finely grated orange rind to the final dough.

The recipe may also be baked in a tray, brownie-like.

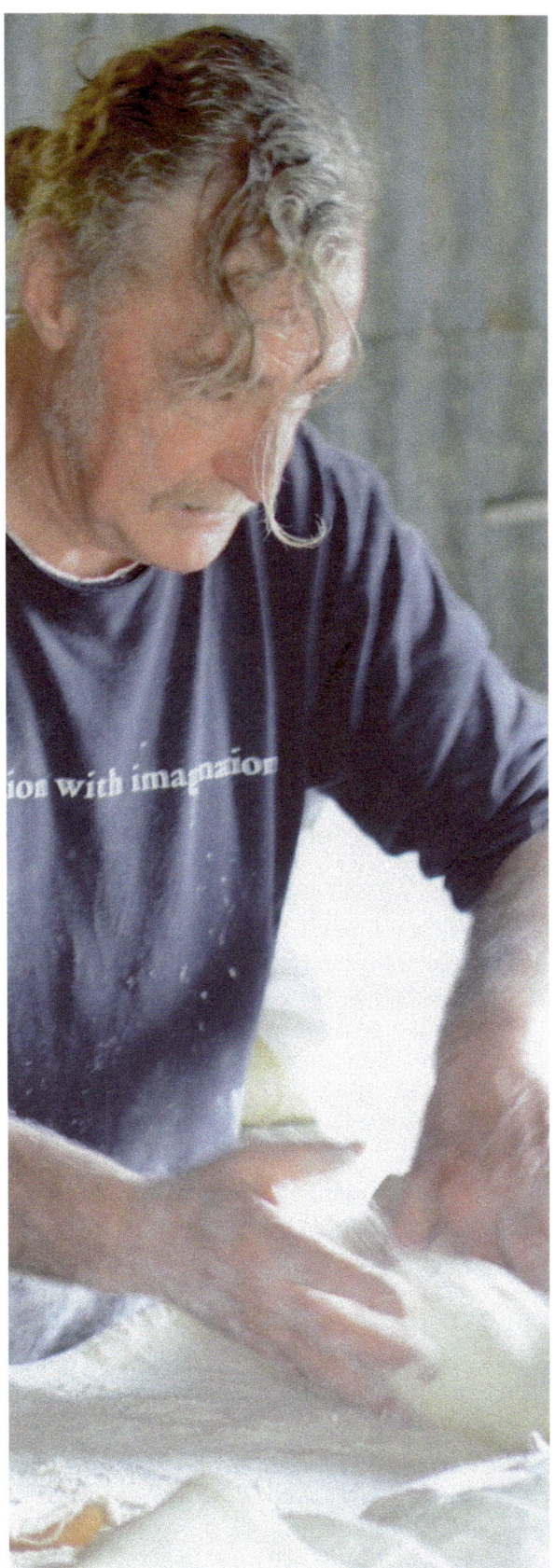

PURI AND PUFFTALOONS

I regularly observed a dough ferment before my eyes in India. Flour, water and the ambient temperature were warm at least, and there was no shortage of bio-activity. This is well recognised in hot countries and enshrined as Jewish dietary law concerning the Passover and the making of ritual matzo bread.

During this religious observance, every conceivable step is taken to ensure that the first bread of the renewal ceremony is absolutely without the corruption of fermentation. It was well recognised that as soon as the dough is made it ferments and so the matzo dough is made from the freshest, just-milled flour and all traces of last year's leaven are thrown away so as not to pollute the air.

The deep-fried flat bread puri is always mentioned in cookery books as "unleavened", yet this only applies to hot countries because the leavening is implicit, usually un-recognised by folk and not commented upon as a method. Making puri in cold weather or in a cold country can be disappointing as the dough will not puff-up nicely when deep-fried, simply because it is not fermented, even slightly, unless the dough is kept, stored or seeded with a sourdough culture.

This may be regarded as more "naturally fermented" than "sourdough", but sometimes, the words get in the way.

Puri and bhatoora are deep-fried thin discs of dough which are a delicate and delicious accompaniment to traditional dishes such as chole (spicy chickpeas, channa), and are often also eaten with fresh curd.

I had such a breakfast early one morning many years ago in rural Myanmar (Burma). Chole (with various names and versions) is one of the best chickpea dishes there is, and this was accompanied by fresh buffalo curd and unrefined sugar.

Puri are made from sifted flour (atta) and bhatoora from white flour (maida). Bhatoora are purposely allowed to ferment and are twice the size (diameter) of poori.

The best dough for making poori is the crusty brown (see p 93) and the white crusty dough for bhatoora (p 91). Allow to ferment for its initial stated proof, and then use for these breads.

Bhatoora method

For bhatoora, when the dough has had its initial ferment, break off egg-size pieces, roll into a ball, allow to relax for a few minutes, and roll into discs, using flour to lightly dust the surface as you roll.

Test the oil by dropping a tiny piece of the dough into it. It should drop to the bottom and immediately rise to the surface of the oil. If the oil is too cool it stays on the bottom, or if too hot it will splatter to the top.

When the oil is at the right temperature, carefully slip in a disc. It will puff nicely, flip it once, the whole frying taking 2 minutes, and then remove to drain on paper or a fine wire drainer. Stack them as you fry.

Use good oil for the frying.... good coconut oil, virgin sesame (best) or mustard (rape) or for sheer deliciousness, good ghee.

Puri method

Puri are smaller than bhatoora, half the size, but the procedure is the same. Puri seem perfect with honey and curd (yoghurt) but accompany savoury dishes as well.

PUFTALOONS ... doughnuts.

Bread dough was often deep-fried in colonial Australia, and elsewhere, and this is the origin of doughnuts. The small pieces of dough, reserved for the baker's breakfast while the bread was rising or baking, swell dramatically when deep-fried. Similarly, pizza, also originated as baker's breakfast while the rest of the dough was rising or baking.

The fried dough pieces were called puftaloons in colonial Australia, in a cracking word play for wicked bakers parodying "pantaloon", a well-known underwear clad comedy figure, as well as slang for puffy ladies underwear. The hot fried dough pieces were usually dredged with sugar while hot or eaten with jam and a cup of tea or coffee.

Puftaloon Method

To make pufftaloons, use the dough when it is well proofed, the white crusty dough (p 91) after 2 hours bulk proof and then 2 hours further proof for example. Break-off small pieces of dough and carefully drop in hot oil without compressing or rolling, the piece should be well aerated. They surface rapidly and resist turning over, so keep them moving with a meshed spoon until lightly coloured and floating. While still hot, roll in panella or rapidura whole cane sugar, or smear with maple syrup, honey jam or your favourite topping,

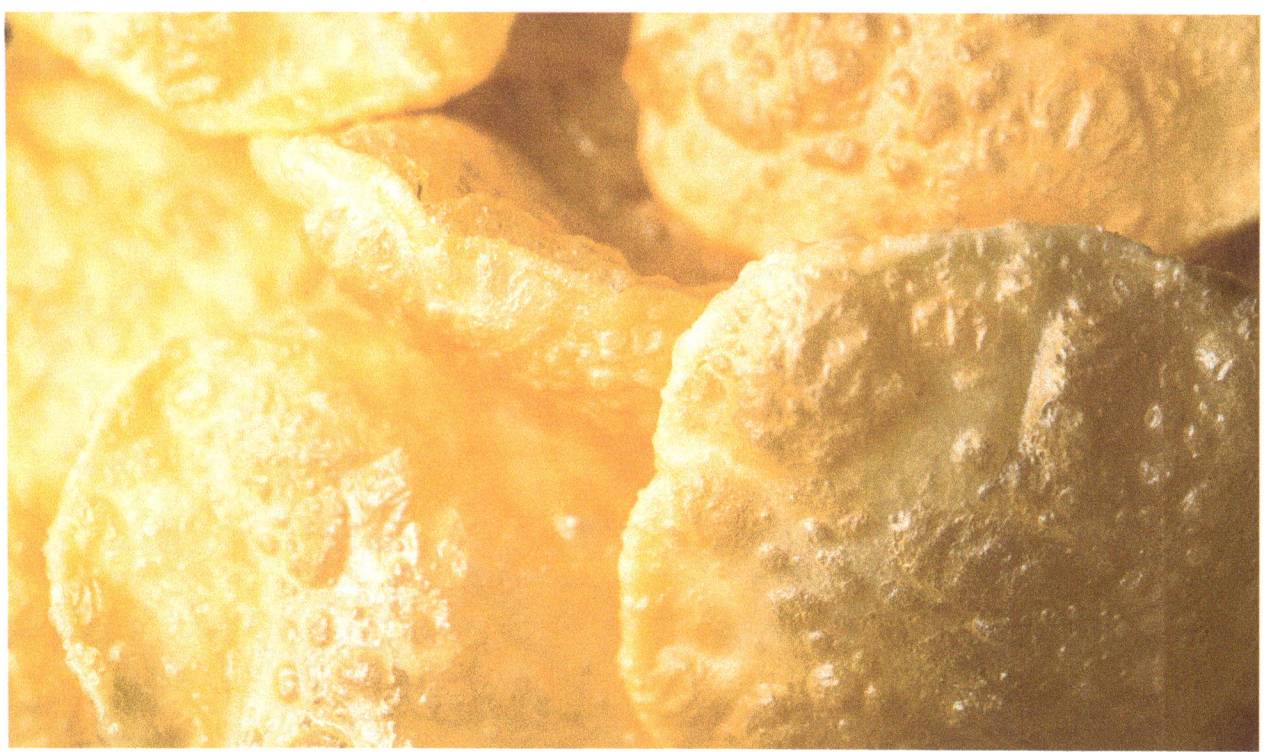

APPLE SOURDOUGH

Ingredients.
- 600 g white (see p 91) or brown (see p 93) dough which has been proofed for 2 hours (white) or 1 hour (brown).
- 250 g panella or rapidura sugar.
- 3 tbsp cinnamon powder - 2 for the apples, 1 for the dough.
- 250 g sultanas.
- 250 g butter/coconut oil or good nut oil.
- 1 tbsp vanilla essence.
- 6 apples.
- Barley malt for glazing.

This is typical of bakers' sweets in the before-patisserie time. Treats such as this were made in large trays and cut into generous slabs, all from simply enriching the bread dough.

The apples may be replaced by other seasonal fruit such as pears apricots or plums, which burst crimson juices and bleed into the dough, or the slice can be infused with spices, dried fruit and or nuts and often jam.

Method
Core the apples and slice through to make thin rounds, mix with 2 tablespoons of the cinnamon and 2 tablespoons of the sugar.

Chop up the dough for easy mixing and add the remaining ingredients except the oil. Mix well, then add the oil and mix to a smooth dough. Cover and let it relax before rolling out or pressing 3 cm thick into an oiled or papered baking tray.

Lay plenty of the heavily cinnamon-ed apples on top. Leave it to proof in a warm spot for 2 hours. It may take longer, wait until well-risen and a bit delicate with the fermentation surging through the core-holes and the apples having sunk slightly.

Bake at 200°C for 30 minutes. While still hot, brush with barley malt.

BROWNIES
Chocolotl Sourdough.

Ingredients.
- 500 g white (see p 91) or brown crusty (see p 93) dough proofed 2 hours (white) or 1 hour (brown).
- 100 g best cacao powder.
- 250 g Panella or rapidura sugar.
- ½ cup softened near-melted butter, ghee or coconut oil or a good nut oil, or melted cacao butter.
- 200 g purple grape juice.
- 2 tbsp, liquid malt extract or pure date syrup or agave syrup.
- 100 g extra flour.
- 4 vanilla pods or 2 tbsp best vanilla essence.

If you have seen the 60's movie, "I love you Alice B Toklas", brownies take on a new hue. Many regular brownies, the "death by chocolate" type are a bit too literal really, the opposite of Alice's.

These brownies were another gift from the muse one sunny day. It is an old bakers-recipe tradition to add cacao to a dough, in the same vein as the apple sourdough, also forgotten due to the puff-pastry and psychedelic-icing psychosis which characterises common bakery items now. It may stretch the definition of brownies a bit, but whatever they are these are great.

Using panella or rapidura sugar gives cacao a wholly new flavour as chocolate. The warm brown whole sugars simply elevate the chocolate-high, harmonising with the cacao and its ancestral friend, (totonac) vanilla. The sourdough fermentation also adds flavour notes which would have been in "chocolotl" from the pulque (maize beer) used in its preparation as a 'gift of the gods'…. like Alice's in a way.

Method
Gently toast/roast the vanilla pods until they waft heavenly aromas, about 10 minutes. Let them cool, remove the hard end nodes, scrape out the seeds and mix them thoroughly with the oil/butter, either in a blender or mortar.

Heat the grape juice and whisk with the cacao, leave it for 30 minutes.

Chop the dough into a dozen pieces for easy mixing. Add the cacao-mix, sugar, malt extract or syrup and extra flour. Mix well then add the oil-vanilla and continue until all is incorporated.

Spread onto an oiled or papered baking tray, about 3 cm thick.

Put it in a big plastic bag and keep in a warm spot. It will rise and be quite delicate in 2-3 hours. Watch, and when it is peaking, obviously well fermented and a bit sponge-like, bake at 200°C for 30 minutes.

It has an unusual, shiny texture.

CHEESE AND ONION ROLLS

Ingredients.
- Double the recipe of Great White sourdough (see p 91).
- 500 g good semi-matured cheese coarsely grated.
- 2 onions finely diced.
- lots of black pepper.
- 1 tsp salt.
- 1 tbsp cumin seeds or 2 tsp of powder.
- 1 egg.

Give the dough 2 hours initial bulk proof, kept warm - it should be well active

Form into a round, rest it 5 minutes, then with a rolling pin and using a little flour for dusting, roll it into a rectangle approximately 29cm wide and 40cm long, and approximately 1 cm thick.

Moisten the edge furthest from you.

Strew the cheese evenly and cover with the onions, sprinkle the salt and cumin and grind on the pepper.

Roll the dough up into a log, beginning with the closest edge. Roll it on to the moistened seam and let it seal. With a sharp knife, cut the log cleanly through each 2 cm to form rounds.

Turn each round onto a well-oiled or papered baking sheet to sit flat almost touching (kissing)

Cover with cloth, then a plastic sheet to keep warm and moist.

These should be well risen in 2 hours, perhaps a little longer.

Make an eggwash by whisking an egg with its volume of water, brush on, and then bake at 250°C for 15 minutes.

I also like to sprinkle Tamari soy sauce on the onions and mix well before adding for a nice savoury touch.

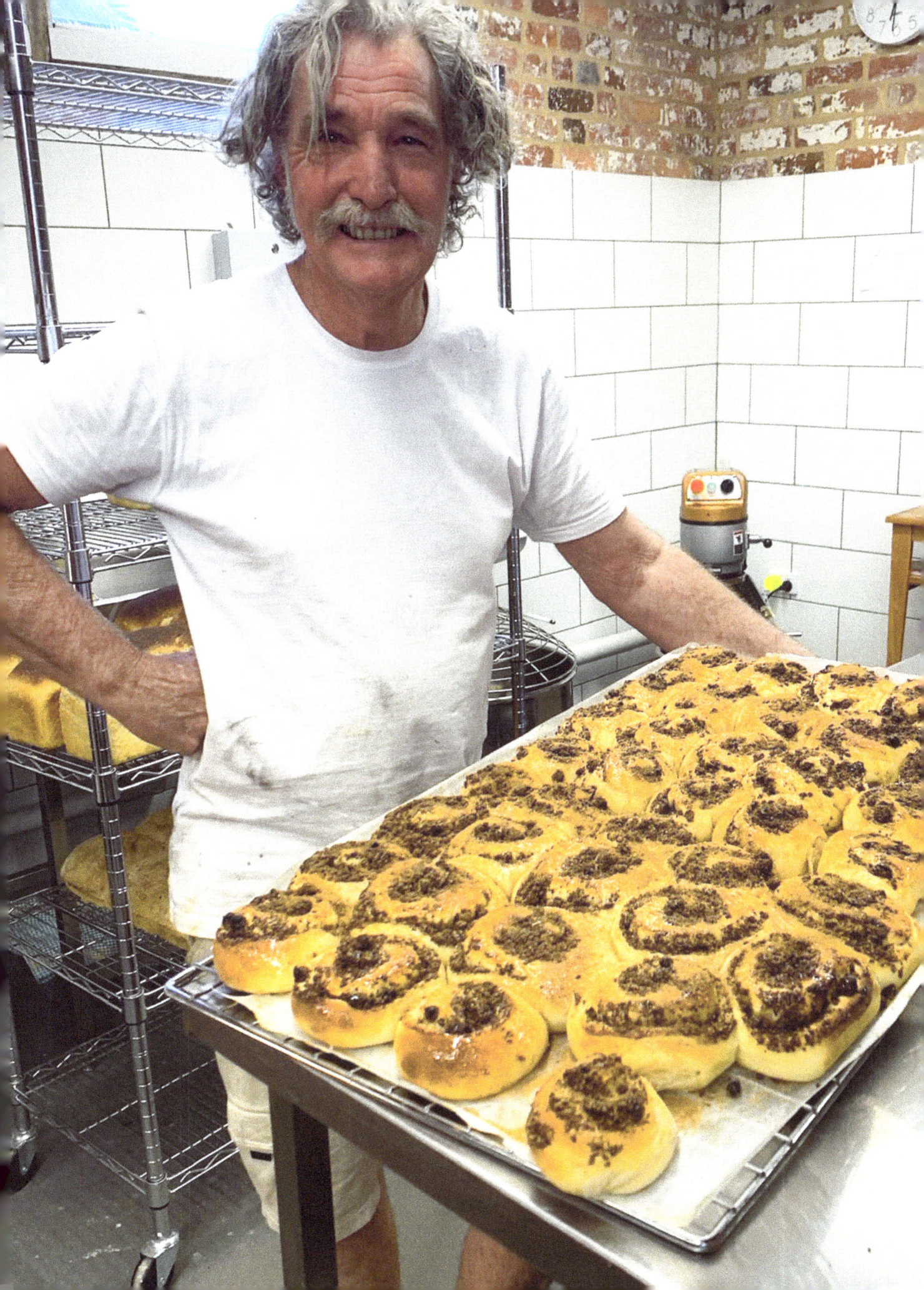

CRUMBLE

The word "crumble" had nothing but a generic meaning to me for years, a type of dessert for example "Apple Crumble" was it. One fine day it hit me......Crumble is derived from Crumb, bread crumb(s), in fact a glaring aspect of language. The ending "le" in English is an adjectival. Thought of this way, Crumble makes absolute sense. It was made with crumb, from leftover and hard bread which was pounded until fine.

In the European "middle ages" the crumb could be sweetened with sugar and spiced with cinnamon or other new spices. Cloves would have gone in with the apples, and often quite a few spices were used.

Butter was still the important nutritious ancient flavour and complement. Bread and butter runs deep, but with the new additions, crumble became a thing.

The modern age brought strange bread which doesn't really crumb and has little flavour, and anyway we were rich enough to throw all the crusts away - increasingly with the bread it came from, and bread consumption plummeted. Crumbles are now made with flour (horrible) and even rolled oats (hippy and good also!).

For homebakers and eateries, this is a good way to use up the leftover crusts. Wholemeal or at least brown bread works best here, as do whole cane juice sugars such as Rapidura or Panella, also muscavado or dark palm/coconut sugar.

Ancient crumbles of superb depth of flavour and fine crumb can be made with honey, barley-malt or date syrup. Using crumb from Emmer bread or Heirloom wheat gives an actual taste of the past which is an insight for we moderns, especially when compared to modern highly sugared and refined sweetness, a benchmark as to how we have changed.

Not especially trying to be Zen, but this is a narrative recipe , there is no metric, which is the history of recipes really. Clearly it is all about getting the right texture.

Method
Crusts may need to be oven dried to crush properly. When dried, either pound or mechwhizz into a coarse meal.

5 cups of my wholemeal crumbs require a cup each of butter and unrefined sugar. Add sugar to the crumbs, mix well and work in or melt-in the butter....which should be unsalted cultured butter. A little fruit juice (from the stewing) may be added to loosen up the texture, but too much will make it hard.

Feel free to add copious amounts of cinnamon or anise seeds or favourite spice, which also depends on the substrate. An apricot crumble demands nutmeg whereas apple crumble demands cinnamon, a peach crumble cassia and a pumpkin crumble may require "pumpkin spice".

The commonest assemblage is to stew or cook or finely slice the fruit. Include the juice from cooking and cover with the crumble. Bake it at 180°C for 20-30 minutes.

Delicious with fresh cream, or custard.

The vegan version is made with coconut oil or even tahina rather than butter.

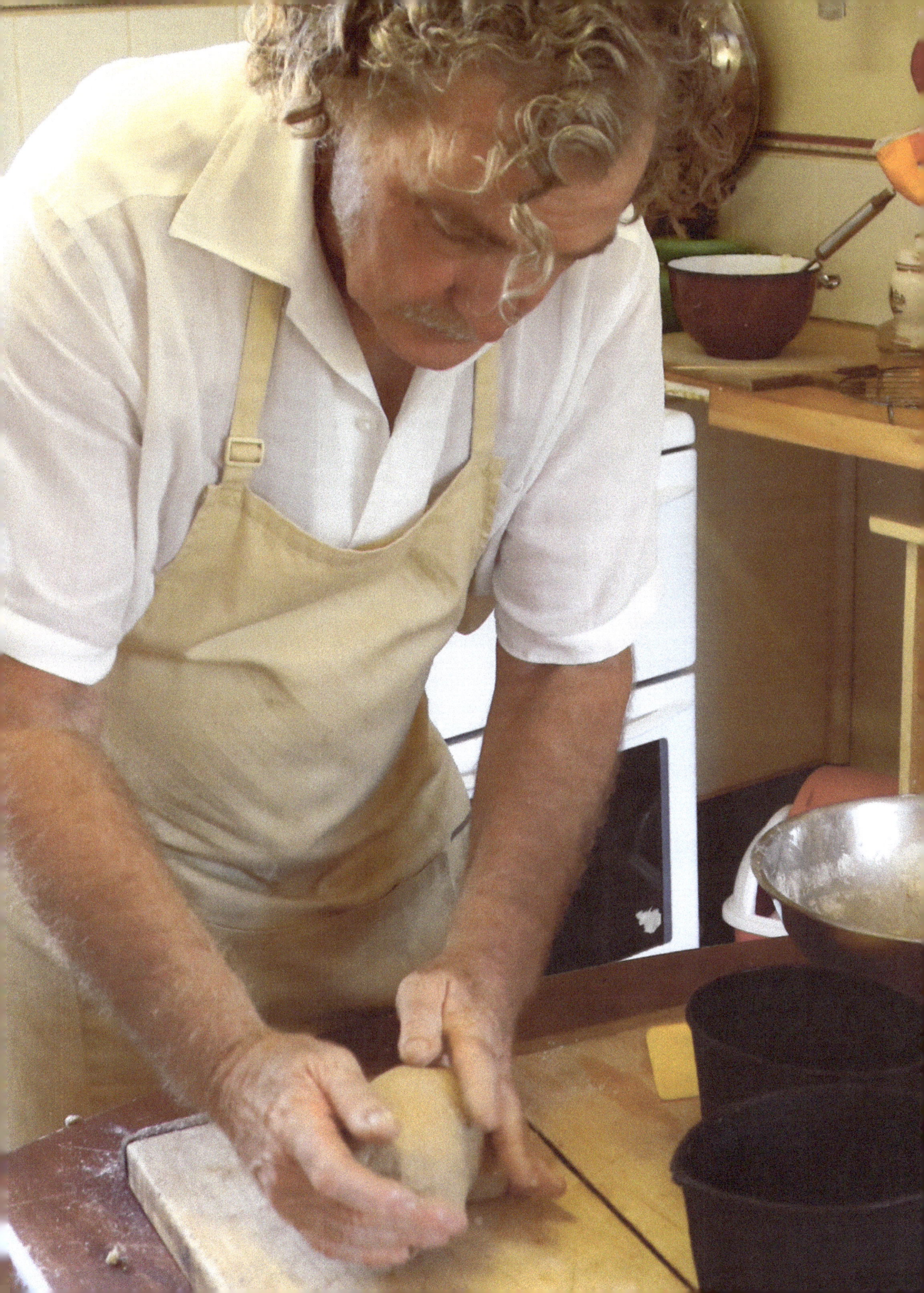

About the Author

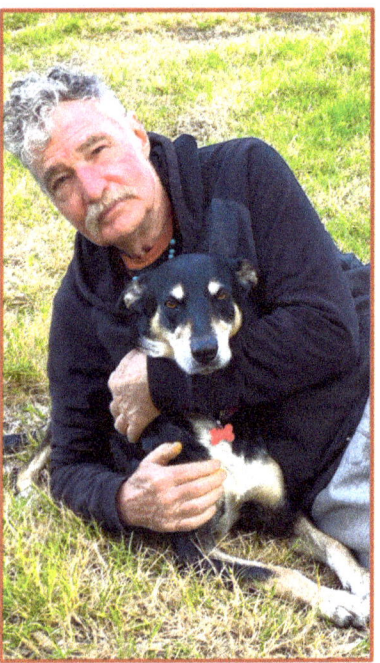

Having pioneered the re-introduction of traditional sourdough bread in the 1970s, John Downes is regarded by many as 'the father of the Australian sourdough bread movement', and in the words of one food critic, a "high priest of sourdough".

John's cooking experience ranges across the culinary spectrum. He has owned several restaurants and bakeries over his career, including some that achieved iconic status in the annals of Australia's food lore. He has worked as Chef for Prime Minister Bob Hawke at the Prime Minister's official residence Kirribilli house in Sydney; as head of the Daylesford Organic Bakery, Oxfordshire, UK; lectured at Ballymaloe Cooking School, in Cork, Eire; and consulted for bakeries in Forest Row, East Sussex; the Shipton Mill, Tetbury, Wiltshire, (the biggest organic flour mill in UK); and Bubiala eco-retreat Tuscany, Italy.

A true polymath, John has an abiding interest in history and culture. Reflecting his belief that many of the forgotten antecedents to modern baking produced deeper flavour and greater wellbeing than modern approaches, John has perfected the art of traditional baking using wood-fired ovens and baking ancient breads using heirloom wheat strains, such as those cultivated by Andrew Forbes (London) and John Letts (Oxfordshire), as well as flours produced by Dayle Lloyd (Eden Valley, WA) and others.

John has a BA and Grad Dip (Gastronomy) from Flinders University in South Australia, has studied Traditional Medicine and Food at Amherst College, (Boston Mass, USA). He is a "Festival Legend" of the Melbourne Food and Wine Festival, and the author of several books on cooking and baking, including the Australian classic Natural Tucker, (Hyland House, 1975).

John lives in South Eastern Queensland, where he continues to bake, research and write on the themes that have guided his career.

Pic: The author and his mate Dookie, 2022.

INDEX

Apple Cider Bread	127
Apple Sourdough	177
Ayurvedic medicine	26
B vitamins	23
Barley	51
Barley and Hazelnut Ring Bread	152
Barley and Oat Ring Breads	151
Barm bread	141
Barmbrack	121
biodynamic	33
Black Bread	110
Boule	95
Bread of the Rings	147
Brownies	178
Buckwheat and Chestnut Ring Breads	154
Cacao Buns	173
Casalinga	91
Cheese and Onion Rolls	179
Chestnut and Azuki Bean Bread	125
Chickpea Manna	159
Chocolotl Sourdough	178
Chocolotls	173
Chorleywood	23
Chorleywood process	29
Coeliac	22
Corn	52
Corn Bread	105
Other "Corn" Breads	107
Crumble	181
Crumpets	152
Crusty Brown Bread	93
Crusty Chestnut Bread	102
Crusty Chickpea Bread	101
Crusty White Sourdough	91
Dayle Lloyd	34
Elizabeth	148
Elizabeth David	23
Emmer Bread	117
Emmer Flatbreads	119
Equipment	57
Bakers "slip"	58
Banneton	59
Cloche	62
Finale	153
Flat breads	33
Flour	36
Buckwheat	54
Cake flour	31
Emmer	27
Kamut	37
khorassan	27, 36–37
roller-milled	33
Rye	36
Sifted flour	35
Sifted stoneground flour	35
spelt	27
Spelt flour	36
stone-ground	34
stoneground flour	35
strong flour	31
Wheat Flours	32
white flour	33
wholemeal flour	36
Ginger Bread	139
gliadin	21
Gluten	21, 31
Bread for Coeliacs	22
coeliac disease	21
Gliadin	21
Gluten intolerance	21
WPD	25
Gluten Free Bread	137
Great White	103
Idli	163
Indian chickpea sourdough bread	162
Indian sourdough	163
Irish Fruit Bread	121
Kuriazukipan	125
Leaven	41
Consistency	45
Flour (for leaven)	45
Ingredients	41
knocking back	44
Making a leaven	41
Preparation for Breadmaking	43
Proof (under/over)	70
Smells	47
Starter	41
Storing and refreshing	43
Temperature	46
The role of the leaven	41
Water (in leaven)	45
Mediterranean diet	19
Method	81
crusty bread template	81
tin bread template	85
Millet	52
Muffyns	155
Must Bread	131
Naan	37
Other grains	53
Oven	65
brick oven	66
pain au levain	35
Pain de Campagne	109
Pane con castagne	102
Pane con ceci	101
Panes Cum Toto	97

Puri and Pufftaloons	175
Purple Wheat and Yellow Corn Bread	135
Rice Bread	137
roller mill	36
Saffron Buns	167
Saffron Oatcakes	154
Salt	55
Sandwich bread	103
Schwarzbrot	110
Shaping	77
sifted-flour-leaven	35
Soca	27
Socca	159
Spelt Bread	111
Steam Bread	171
Steam Buns	171
Technique	69
Temperature	71
Texture	74
Time	69
Tropical Fruit Bread	120
Uni Appam	153
Water	55
Western pattern diet	25
Wheat	31
Canadian hard wheat	26
durum wheat	37
Dwarf wheat	27
Einkorn	38
Emmer	37
hard wheat	31
heirloom wheat	27
Heritage Wheat	38
Ukrainian hard wheat	26
Wheat in diet	26
Wheat Ring Breads and crumpets	152
Wholemeal wheat bread	97
Yeoman's Loaf	109

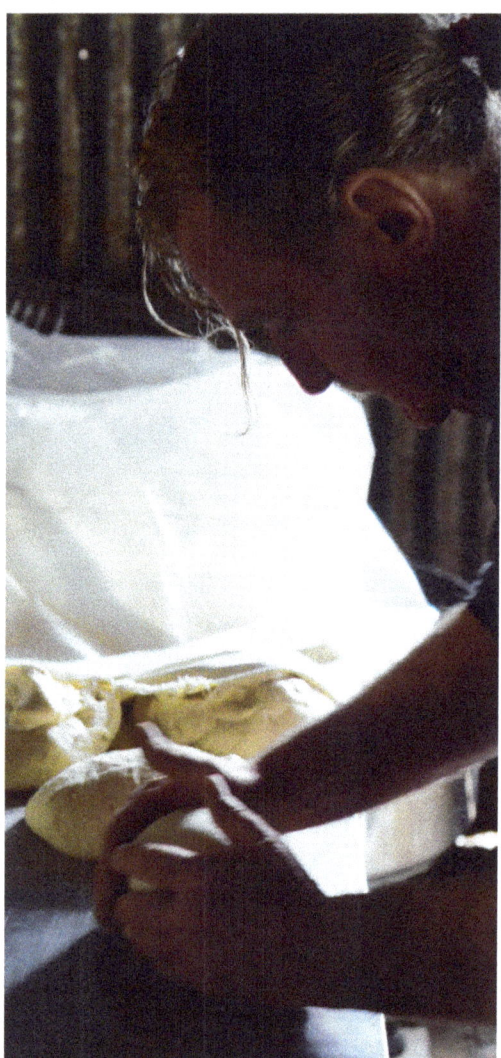